flirtexting®

revised edition

PRAISE FOR FLIRTEXTING

"Flirting via text message—or 'Flirtexting'—is a must in today's dating world." **—AM New York**

"Every girl has a great flirtexting story! And if you don't, you will after reading this." **—Kristen Cavallari, Actress**

"A modern day guide on how to use different forms of technology to find a guy (or two)." **—Star Magazine**

"Oh, the agony of dating in the digital age. How long do you wait before responding to his text? What does it mean when she doesn't text you back right away? How should you reply when she asks what you're doing tonight? The questions are potentially endless. Fortunately, flirtexting experts Olivia Baniuszewicz and Debra Goldstein—who literally wrote the book on flirtexting—are here to save the day." **—Huffington Post**

"If only poor Mary, Drew Barrymore's character in *He's Just Not That Into You,* had a copy of *Flirtexting* on hand to help her navigate the world of online dating, she might not have ended up with a schlep like the ScarJo-besotted Kevin Connolly." **—ELLE Canada**

"Olivia and Debra who wrote the book *Flirtexting* which btdubbs is so cute and LOL, you guys will love it I promise" **—Ross Mathews, *Chelsea Lately* and HelloRoss.com**

"Debra Goldstein and Olivia Baniuszewicz are known as 'The Digital Abby's' of the 21st Century." —*Lifestyle* **from Yahoo Canada**

"Liv and Deb know so much about texting with dudes that I've had to destroy my phone. Twice." —**Ben Lerer, Founder of Thrillist.com**

"*Flirtexting: How to Text Your Way to His Heart* will not only get you a date, but it'll also make you LOL." —*Redeye*

"Arguing that 'boys text; therefore girls need to know how to flirtext,' first-time authors (and, presumably, BFFAEs) Goldstein and Baniuszewicz show the next generation of single women how to entertain suitors with the art of text message flirtation. With this guide at hand, young singles won't be at a loss for words—at least until their next F2F (face to face) encounter." —*Publisher's Weekly*

flirtexting®
revised edition

how to text your way

into his heart

Olivia Baniuszewicz **and** Debra Goldstein

Foreword by E. Jean Carroll

Skyhorse Publishing

Skyhorse Publishing books may be purchased in bulk at special discounts for sales promotion, corporate gifts, fund-raising, or educational purposes. Special editions can also be created to specifications. For details, contact the Special Sales Department, Skyhorse Publishing, 307 West 36th Street, 11th Floor, New York, NY 10018 or info@skyhorsepublishing.com.

Skyhorse® and Skyhorse Publishing® are registered trademarks of Skyhorse Publishing, Inc.®, a Delaware corporation.

www.skyhorsepublishing.com

10 9 8 7 6 5 4 3 2 1

Library of Congress Cataloging-in-Publication Data is available on file.

ISBN: 978-1-62087-183-6

Printed in China

Wardrobe courtesy of INTERMIX.

To my parents, whose inspiring 40-year marriage
started with handwritten love letters,
whatever those are.
—Debra

To my mom, whose advice will
always be the first and last I'll take.
—Olivia

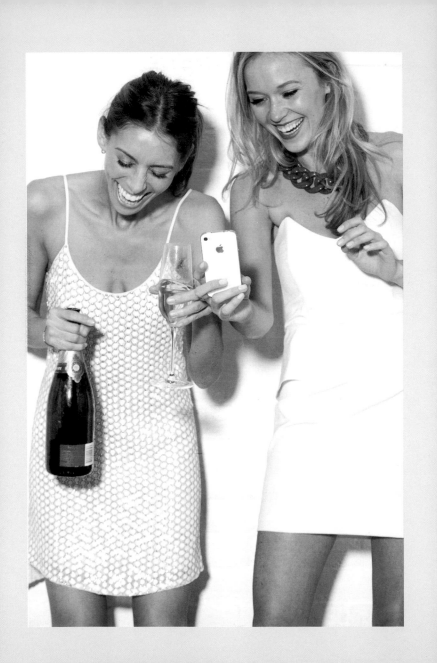

Contents

· · · · · · · · · · · · · · · · · · · ·

PART ONE:

why text?

· · · · · · · · · · · · · · · · · · · ·

FOREWORD

Debra Goldstein and Olivia Baniuszewicz are the Hemingway and Fitzgerald of texting. As two of the greatest texting stylists in the English language, they know how to bewitch a man right out of his brains.

Indeed, Debra and Olivia know better than anyone the power of making a man wait—of tormenting him! Vexing him! Driving him mad with anticipation! And they show you about 500 different ways to do this with Facebook, text, and email. Here's one of my favorites: *"If he texts you, then the ball is in your court and you hold the power. We recommend you try and hold onto that power for as long as your manicured hands can."*

Olivia and Debra not only give you witty responses to every conceivable text or Facebook message a chap can send you—they give you something a thousand times more important: The age-old secrets of allure. (And these ladies know more about allure than Aphrodite.)

When you've devoured this book—and it goes down like a sparkling Bellini—you'll understand why this preface is so brief. One of Debra and Olivia's rules is: You should say just enough to make the reader want more.

E. Jean Carroll
Elle Magazine

FLIRTEXTING STYLE QUIZ

. . . .

What Type of Flirtexter Are You?

Everyone has their own flirting style that trans-lates into their flirtexting technique. Knowing how you communicate your romantic interest via flirtext can help you improve your chances at love. Circle your answer to each texting scenario to see what kind of flirtexter you are.

Scenario 1: He sends you an "accidental" blank text. You flirtext back…

a) "Glad we caught up. Good talk."

b) "Your phone must miss me."

c) "Tell your phone to stop playing hard to get."

d) "Heyyyy! I think you just texted me but it's blank. What's up?"

Scenario 2: He sends this evidently drunk, LNBT (late night booty text): "Whyy dont u commee ovr?" You flirtext back . . .

a) "Sorry, got a few other offers with less mis-spellings."

b) "Flattered, I'm sure. How about a hangover curing brunch instead?"

c) "Wow, is this what it feels like to be wooed by you? I can't wait to see what tomorrow brings."

d) "On my way. See you soon babe!!"

Scenario 3: He texts, "You missed the best night last night," meanwhile he never invited you out. You flirtext back…

a) "Cool. My invite clearly got lost in the mail."

b) "Couldn't have been THAT much fun without moi."

c) "Clearly, you aren't aware of what I did last night . . . but I'm so glad you enjoyed yours as well."

d) "But not as good as mine: Ryan Gosling on demand with a touch of mint chocolate ice cream."

Scenario 4: He texts: "You thinking about me a lot?" You flirtext back…

a) "Meh…"

b) "Is this your way of letting me know you're thinking about me without actually saying it? You're cute."

c) "I'd say maybe 5 percent of the day. The rest is split among my other suitors."

d) "Duh. Like every second of every day."

Scenario 5: He responds to your phone call with a "What's up?" text. You flirtext back . . .

a) "The person you have reached is allergic to getting texts in response to their calls. Please try again."

b) "Your voice is way sexier than your texts. I'd consider rethinking that choice."

c) "The Sky? Call me back when you get a minute."

d) "Ouch. Why didn't you pick up?"

Scenario 6: His concerning text: "I feel like we're moving in different directions." You flirtext back...

a) "Sorry I'm not an ambi-turner like you . . . I can't turn left." (Zoolander movie quote!)

b) "Cool, I get it. But can we at least chat on the phone before pulling the trigger? Don't like having these types of convos via text."

c) "Is it too late to say I, too, love watching sports, eating wings, and drinking beer?"

d) "What did I do wrong? Tell me and I'll try to change."

Scenario 7: His text: "Sorry I never responded to your text Friday night. My phone broke and I just got it fixed." You flirtext back . . .

a) "I sent you a text Friday?"

b) "Great. Apologize to your mom for all my concerning calls on Saturday."

c) "Ah, the ole "my phone broke excuse." I'll give you half credit for that one. More creativity next time."

d) "No worries. I just thought you were no longer into me!"

SCORING

Mostly A's — Sassy You're confident, smart, and always looking for an "LOL." Your comedic relief is refreshing and guys see you as a challenge. Others, however, might take your sarcasm as a sign you're not into them. Be aware of this and try to let your sassy guard down a bit. If you do, be prepared for them to keep coming back for more!

Mostly B's — Flirty You're a sweet flirt who lets guys know how you feel without being too forward. You understand their needs and your flirtexts are light and fun. Guys see you as the "girl-next-door," they always want you around.

Mostly C's — Straight shooter You tell it like it is and refuse to play games. Guys respect your honesty but can also find it intimidating. It'll take a guy with confidence and a backbone to handle your straight up approach.

Mostly D's — Fast Track Jane Playing hard to get is a foreign concept to you as you're on the fast track to settling down. You make yourself available whenever he asks and dream of being swept off your feet. Your fantasy of finding a white knight is unrealistic and will create problems for you down the road (if it hasn't already).

What type of flirtexter are you? _____

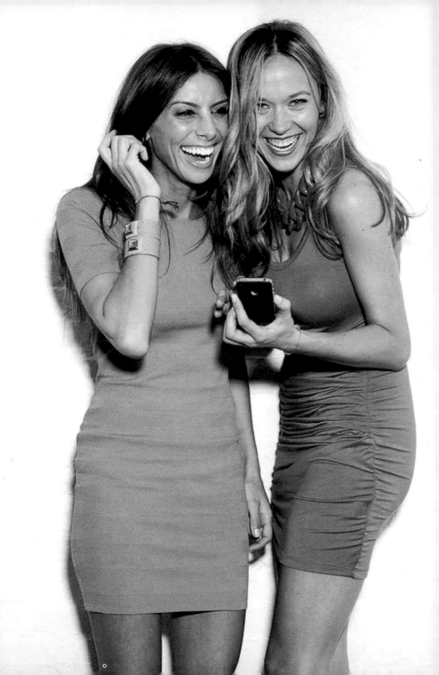

PART ONE:

why text?

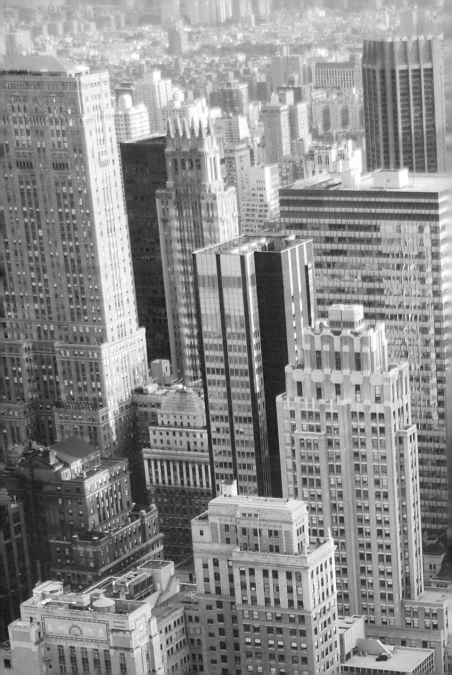

TEXT IN THE CITY

"I'll do whatever it takes to get girls to go
out with me. If the new thing is wearing
a bag over my head, then that's what I'm
gonna do. Right now it happens to be
texting. So I'm all over it." —Eric

Recently, we were having drinks in the city with a
few of our girlfriends when Olivia received a text
message from her current crush. We became instantly
excited and screamed for her to read it out loud. After
analyzing every last word, we each shared our brilliant
thoughts on how Olivia should respond. We put lots
of time and energy into creating something delicious
. . . and finally came up with the best possible text.
And, as an added touch, we delayed sending the text
for two hours. The result: an immediate response and,
soon after, an official date invite! Believe it or not, you

have the secret weapon in your hand and it can lead to whatever kind of relationship you want with the guy on the other end—friendship, innocent flirtation, possible hook-up, or romance. Your cell phone has become the most widely used tool in scoring that hot date. The strategic use of text messaging in dating is called *flirtexting*, or *flirting over text*.

> **A Flirtext is any text message sent between you and someone you would like to date or are currently dating, composed of flirty, witty banter that helps build a connection.**

We're single, independent, women, gallivanting about the social scene of NYC. We're flirts who love to go out and enjoy meeting interesting people.

At the start, we had the same questions (Does he really like me if he's texting and not calling?) and concerns (Is it too soon to text back?) as you. Through the surplus of single and suitable men that our city has so graciously left on our doorstep, we've been able to play the field while using the logic of trial and error to create our method. We gained confidence with each and every text we received and sent, leading to more date invites than days in a week.

Now, flirtexting has become the *new first step* in dating. It's time to upgrade to that unlimited texting plan and improve your typing skills. In the following chapters, you have tried-and-true information, perfected in the finest dating capital in the nation, New York City. Whether it's "Mr. Right" or "Mr. Right Now" you're pining after, flirtexting will help you get what you want. **In *Flirtexting*, we provide the ultimate guide to wooing your guy over text.** After using the skills taught in this book, you will have your latest prospect in the palm of your hand—literally. Message received?

When done strategically, texting can help you get a date, and potentially a boyfriend. Exactly what you write back and when you write back will determine which direction your relationship will go.

Flirtexting is an efficient means for guys and girls to explore one another's feelings and see if there's mutual attraction. If the response is positive, and you both like what you read, you'll eventually take the next steps: Facebook friends, phone call, date, meet the parents, accept Facebook friend requests from his parents, the usual. To get to that point, you must first impress each other through text. This book gives you the skills you need in order to feel prepared and

"Hi. Want to Grab a Drink 2nite?"

Um, hello! Is this supposed to be charming? If he really cared, wouldn't he call or ask me out in person? Have you turned down tons of decent guys just because they were texting and not calling? Well, so did we, gals . . . so did we. Until now! We stopped fighting it and figured out how to make flirtexting work for us, and so can you.

texting tip

confident when pressing send. If you play your texts right (and follow our suggestions), you'll ultimately learn how to seduce the man of your dreams, through text.

Our motivation for writing this book came from our girlfriends' overzealous efforts to hookup with their Prince Charmings, fall in love, and get married. Single women everywhere have worried about this for ages. Societal pressures to get married and start a family are still very present today, leading to the notion that there must be something wrong with you if you don't settle down by a certain age. Our take on this is to understand that your time will come, and realize that falling in *true* love cannot be forced. More often than not, love arrives unexpectedly. Therefore, it's time to take a chill pill (literally, if psychiatric need be), work on ourselves first, and allow Mr. Right to find us. Trust that in due time, he will. It's inevitable.

> **Fast Track Jane: The insecure girl (in all of us), who at times lets the overbearing societal pressures of settling down get the best of her, causing her to act in unflattering ways that can turn guys off.**

When working on our relationships, we can sometimes lose sight of ourselves. The fight for love has led

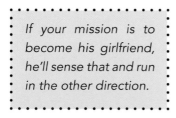

If your mission is to become his girlfriend, he'll sense that and run in the other direction.

girls to move cross-country to follow their latest prospect, act/dress/speak like an ex-girlfriend, take an interest in deep-sea fishing (despite being deathly

texting tell-all

Deep Thoughts by Deb & Liv

There's a large misconception that we need to be with a partner in order to be happy. This innate pressure many of us carry has led girls to desperately seek someone, *anyone,* in the name of love. Well, we've got news, "desperate" is not the look you want to be sporting when searching for love. *The best advice we've ever received was to become the person you want to marry.* Ultimately, you're the only one that can make yourself happy. Strive to have all the qualities you look for in a partner so that you are complete without needing to depend on another person. Don't look for someone to fill a void in yourself. The goal is not to complete each other, but rather to complement one another so that you can grow together. Work on being happy with yourself first. Then your relationships will flourish, because you stopped depending on someone else for your happiness. This is the key to a happy you and a lasting relationship.

We've found these books to be helpful on the journey of self-exploration:

The Four Agreements
The Secret
5 Languages of Love

afraid of water), and even turn Republican. Undoubtedly, the dedication to finding love is there; however, the pressure to get that ring and settle down can become so overpowering that sometimes girls don't realize that their attempt makes them come across looking transparently desperate.

We've seen the gorgeous and talented get rejected, the sweet and smart turn needy. We've watched the independent and fun suddenly turn dependent and pushy, and then get dumped . . . at the altar. In due time, the women who attracted these men in the first place disappears, and the men shortly thereafter. Sadly, these girls more often than not become the rejectees and not the rejectors. Knowing that these women really are quite the catch, we don't like what we see.

It saddens us to see our beautiful, smart, remarkably witty girlfriends scare guys off due to their unconscious ploys to make them commit. Therefore, we found it necessary to eradicate any "desperate girl syndrome" by teaching confidence through text. *There's no better way to hook a guy than through a witty flirtext.* Texting has invaded our lives and our little black books. We've embraced it and it's done wonders to our dating lives, and now it's your turn! Consider this our gift to you: intervention for love. Ladies, allow us show you how to text your way into his heart.

Standing in for all the girls we mentioned above, and the societal fast track they're pressured to be on, we'll reference them as a character named Jane. Jane is desperate to find love. Jane is every girl's faulty side when she's playing the field of love. Don't be Jane.

Jane's lame. It is important, however, to acknowledge Jane's presence, as it is vital in acknowledging our own faults and addressing them head-on. Jane is meant to be a reflection of our social imperfections and conundrums of dating. She will be your "what not to do" girl. Learn from Jane's mistakes. There are many vital lessons to be learned.

texting tell-all

See How We Came Across the Beauty of the Text and Made It Work for Us.

"It's not a southern thing,
it's a Deb thing." —Debra

Growing up in the South has preconditioned me to a dating etiquette that is as traditional as it gets. I expect guys to call me first, open my door, make the first move, and laugh at all my jokes. (Okay this may not be a Southern thing ... it's a Deb thing). When this doesn't happen, I can't say I'm not disappointed. Although I've become more forgiving toward guys as I've gotten older and moved away from the South, when it comes down to basic dating courtesy, I won't budge.

So you can imagine my frustration when guys began asking me out over text. I kept thinking to myself that *my* Mr. Right would never text message me out on a first date. Being on the slightly stubborn side, I held strong for a while and turned down any guy who asked me out over text.

This went on for some time and consequently my dance card became less full. It wasn't until a cutie with true potential came along—a guy who, like most, just loves to text—that I broke this little rule of mine. Then I cut the next guy some slack, and so on and so forth.

Cut to … three years later … and we're writing a book about how great texting and dating is.

texting tell-all

> "I got asked to my prom
> via text message!" —Olivia

It was my junior year in high school. JD sent me a text one day after school. JD's ID? He was my friend and a hot senior guy whom sources had revealed had a mini-crush on yours truly.

The texting went back and forth as we reviewed each other's days and sports practices, which led to:

"Are you going to prom?"

"Yes, obviously."

"Do you want to go together? It'll be fun."

"Really? Over text JD?"

"Is that a yes?"

Even though I had seen JD about two hours earlier, he neglected to hold this convo face-to-face (F2F). Needless to say, he ended up escorting me to my much-hyped prom. Being a girl who loves traditional approaches, this invitation left me somewhat embarrassed and confused. After all, my date put as much thought into asking me as Kim Kardashian put into her marriage. I am pleased to report we rocked the prom despite that shaky start.

"I love flirtexting because through my digital 'game' I can quickly establish the upper hand." —**Nick**

WE DATE THEREFORE WE TEXT

Somewhere between the time *90210* went off the air and came back on (with a new cast), we came to terms with what we knew all along but weren't ready to admit: Texting has become the *new first step* in dating, and it's here to stay. Sadly, we had to say *buh-bye* to our traditional, and now outdated, way of thinking. We have now learned to embrace flirtatious texts and the relationships that they breed. Upon finally recognizing the undeniable power of text, our phone simultaneously became our BFF and our dating tool. We soon realized that texting really isn't all that bad. In fact, it's pretty amazing.

[**Communi-dating:** **How we date through our various forms of digital and wireless communication, i.e., text, BBM, e-mail, phone, Facebook, Match.com, etc.**]

Our hectic schedules benefit from a shortcut as often as possible. Between having a productive day's

> *Draft a text like a Post-it note . . . quick and memorable.*

work, hitting the gym, eating dinner, watching *The Bachelor*, and going to bed, it's difficult to reconnect with those near and dear to us. Thankfully, technology has been able to keep up with our busy lives. If we don't have time to call, no big deal; we can text. Texting takes ¼ the amount of time, and allows us to connect with more people than, say, a phone call.

Perhaps the name explains it all: SMS stands for Short Message Service and it speaks volumes about our generation; one that likes to keep it short and to the point. UG8TIT? When given the opportunity, we'd so much rather say it in four words or less. Look at it this way: If you're given a large piece of paper to write a short message, you will feel pressure to write a lot and divulge unnecessary details. But if you're given a Post-it note to write that same message, you'll write only what

texting tip

As Communication Majors in College, we learned that, invariably, the way a message is sent is more important than the content of the message itself. Due to its informality, texting has allowed us to become more approachable and open with our feelings toward one another. The low-risk, no-strings-attached approach that texting provides has given us a newfound confidence, which we in turn use to our advantage.

you must—*a short message.* Plus, with ADD (Attention Deficit Disorder) affecting 99 percent of our peers (or so it seems), text allows us to get straight to the point: "Fro yo vs ice cream throwdown—are you game?"

Little Black Book

The little black book used to be a small, usually black, notebook in which guys and dolls would store names, numbers, and notes of everyone they've dated, are dating, or would like to date. Frequently you would find little stats about each person next to their name. For instance, "Keith from New York: likes Polish food" or "Rich: Great kisser, big jerk" … you get the idea. How clever and handy.

With convenience and speed on its side, the cell phone has taken over the function of the little black book. You can still make those same notes as you would before, like "Dave: Met at Sarah's bday. Sooo hot. Want to date!!" Only now, you can also use it to contact hot Dave with the touch of a button. This slick, mini device stores not only our contacts, but our stories and secrets, too. Plus, cell phones are digital, so you can back them up and never have to worry about losing anyone's information. **The little black book has gone wireless and our social calendars have blossomed because of it.**

[
Nomophobia: Also known as "no mobile-phone phobia" is the act of feeling anxious and tense when one is out of reach of their phone.
]

Why We Love Flirtexting

1. *An outlet for mass flirting!*

    If you're anything like us, you speak in flirt! Texting allows you to flirt on a totally different level than before. You can text with many guys at once and only your cell knows about it. If there are three guys you've been crushing on, text them all to see what they're doing and hope the one you like most asks you out!

2. *Helps eliminate social barriers such as shyness.*

    This is your chance to experiment with being more open about your feelings in a controlled environment. Text is taken a lot more lightly than a phone call, e-mail, or F2F (face-to-face) conversation. Therefore, it allows you to take more chances in life and in love. Use text as a testing ground to say things you might be hesitant to say in person. If it ever backfires, you can always just say that you were only kidding. Did he not hear the sarcasm in your text?

3. *Girls can ask guys out . . . and not feel weird about it.*

    In the olden days, or B.T. (before text), it was quite unusual for a gal to ask a guy out. Since texting wasn't around during *The Rules* conversation, no clear-cut "rules" were ever set. Text has created a loophole to our moms' old-fashioned approach of waiting for him to ask us out first, while keeping our code of etiquette above board. So if there's a cute young lad you're crusing on . . . text away!

4. *Makes rejection easier to handle.*

    If a guy is calling you and you just aren't feeling it, texting him back instead of calling delivers the message, and avoids the awkward rejection. That makes it easier on you both and will hopefully save the friendship. This also applies for the opposite of this scenario. If you text a guy and he doesn't write you back, aka radio silence, then nine out of ten times, he's just not that into you. Ugh, the perils of dating.

5. *Fits into our fast-paced lives.*

    Texting makes it easy to keep in touch in a quick and efficient way. When we don't have time to pick up the phone and call, a short text gets the job done easily. Making a phone call wastes crucial getting ready time, but sending a text to let him know you're running late for your date is completely sufficient.

Why Guys Love Flirtexting

- "I love flirtexting because it gets the first date B.S. out of the way. So when we finally meet it's on!!" —Brett

- "I love flirtexting because you can have eight convos going on at once and it's not like you're dating all eight girls at the same time. It's a thrill." —Sebastian

- "I don't love flirtexting, I lust it." —Gene

Texting by Date of Birth

Texting is subjective. It's what you want it to be. Think of texting as the Op-Ed section of *The New York Times*, open to your participation however much or little you want. Each age group has its own comfort level and willingness to engage. The groups are divided into three brackets that significantly differentiate one from the other. However, there's one tie that binds us all together: **We date, therefore we text!!**

Here's where you stand:

1. *Late Teens/Early Twenties*

   You're a Starbucks-sipping, Converse-sporting, sexually charged teenager with the latest cell phone. When we were your age we passed folded notes; you're doing the same but with text messages. Teens seem to be the most savvy when it comes to techno-relating because they started young. Texting is your world.

2. *Mid-twenties/Late Twenties*

   When you began dating, guys called to ask you out. You have since segued into dating in today's flirtexting era. Therefore, you're a bit unsure how the rules have changed since texting took over the courtship. At first, you told everyone you hated flirtexting and insisted guys call. But then you realized texting is *ah-mazing*, because it's a huge timesaver and an outlet for major flirting. Twenty-somethings actually have the best of both worlds because you've adopted texting as your new go-to for dating, but also know when it's appropriate to call.

3. *Thirties and Up*

You thought texting was just a way to relay information, i.e., to tell someone you are on your way or to give directions. You believed that e-mailing was the ticket that led to that phone conversation. But then you met a hottie at a bar and he asked you out via text. And you thought, "I could have fun with this!" You are confident, self-sufficient, and know where you are heading in life. You know what you want and how to express it. Texting is the perfect tool for you to take what you know and apply it through flirtexting.

An Ode to *The Rules*

In order to understand our approach, you must first understand where we are coming from. The two of us are "*Rules* Girls." If you aren't already aware of what being a *Rules* Girl means, it means playing a little hard to get, to get what you want. By not giving away too much at first, you leave him wanting more. *The Rules* is a book that teaches you that, through phone conversations and in person, the more mystery you create and maintain, the more interested your crush will be. In *Flirtexting,* we teach you how to obtain that same sought-after attention, via text.

With technology rapidly becoming the means by which we communi-date, ultimately *The Rules* have to be adjusted to today's times. If we want to remain on top of our dating game, we need to keep up and adapt. We find it necessary to apply these old rules to modern times. For instance, *The*

Our book is for anyone who is single with a cell phone. It is targeted toward girls, because—let's be honest—guys don't like to work on relationships! But, we know they'd be tempted to sneak a peek if this guide were sitting on their girlfriend's coffee table. As a kind gesture to the men we text, we unveil our likes and dislikes throughout the book so that they know just how to text their way into our phones and, eventually, our hearts.

Rules state: "Always end phone calls first." We agree with this rule and think it's essential you apply it to flirtexting conversations as well. For instance, if you're having a flirtexting convo with a current crush, *it's best to let his text be the last sent*. This also applies for starting up flirtexting conversation; you should *allow him to start more of the conversations than you*. It's about him pursuing you and not the other way around. You want his word to be the last, so he's left wanting more of you and your conversation. We consider this a *texting cliffhanger*—he'll want to fill his desire to communicate with you more.

We truly believe that *The Rules* will always be that by which we live and date. However, today we live in a flirtexting world, so it's importatnt to keep the old rules, but learn to apply the new ones so you don't fall behind.

The Usual Suspects

With its non-threatening approach, texting has made flirting with tons of guys more accessible. It's easier and quicker to weed through the many guys you have a crush on and see whether you want to take that relationship to the next level.

If you're single, this is who you are flirtexting …

The Guy(s) of the Moment	This is the one you are currently dating or entertaining the thought of dating, and your flirtexts usually consist of funny, light jabs to one another. You're building a bond that'll lead to a series of dates and eventually, if you deem worthy, a potential relationship. You are very careful when composing your flirtexts to him and usually find it necessary to consult a friend. (Totally normal and cute.)

An Old Boyfriend	Texting is the perfect way to keep in touch with old boyfriends, especially when you need a little boost of self-confidence. Your relationship with this old BF ended amicably, and even if he's in a new relationship now, you still keep in touch by flirtexting. There's an undeniable spark you two share, and you like to see if it's still there from time to time. Your flirtexts are commonly reflective of the type of things you said to one another when you were in a relationship.

Your "Guy Friend"	This is one of your close friends who you either hooked up with many moons ago or swear to everyone that you are "just friends" despite the fact it's obvious there's sexual tension between the two of you. Your flirtexts consist of playful teasing and mentions of how much you miss each other when you're not together. Take a tip from the theme in *When Harry Met Sally*: Men and women can't ever just be friends because the sex part always gets in the way.

A Guy You Briefly Dated	This relationship may have been as brief as a spring break hook-up, but there's no denying sometimes it just feels good to flirtext with an old flame. He may live far away now, or perhaps there just wasn't enough chemistry for it to work. Regardless, it's always fun to have flirtatious banter with him when you get the urge.

texting tell-all

Volleying for Love

Our friend Jill was playing ping-pong with some friends one night. She spotted a certifiable PBF playing at the table next to hers so she decided to "accidentally" hit the ball onto his table. Whoopsie! The night ended with them exchanging numbers. The next day she received the following text from him: "Nice game Jill. Your backhand could use some work though. When do we rematch?" Score! Not only was she impressed by his pong game, but judging by his clever and charming text, she was sure he was a winner off the table, too. Her flirtext response read a little something like this: "Actually, I let you win . . . My trainer doesn't allow me to play with amateurs but I made an exception for you. Rematch next weekend."

Cut to one year later, and there were ping-pong tables set up at Jill and Matt's wedding reception. Matt finally found his match in Jill, on and off the court. Jill says it was their first exchange of awesome texts that set the tone for their happily ever after.

Here's the Point of Your Initial Response Text:

1. Confirm your interest in him.

2. Make him smile, laugh, and blush. Do all three and you're a sure thing.

3. Reflect your personality: funny, flirty, sarcastic, etc.

4. Out-do his initial text. You may not always hit the mark, but at least shoot for the stars. If his initial text was boring, then you have little work cut out for you.

5. Get a date invite.

Your Second First Impression

Your initial text is one of the most important flirtexts you'll send. It's so important, we call it *your second first impression*. You can tell a lot about a person by what they text. The only way for him to get to know you at this early stage is through your texts. Therefore, the better you text the more he will like you. It's as simple as that. In Jill and Matt's case, they were able to reconfirm their mutual attraction and similar sense of humor through their flirtexts.

Your initial response text is a chance to show your degree of interest and showcase your personality. If his initial text hits it out of the park and you like him, you should respond with equal or greater enthusiasm and awesomeness.

Your initial response text is a chance to flash your playing cards so he knows what he's up against. When a guy nails a great text, surprise him by throwing back something even better. By outdoing his initial text, he'll become intrigued and come back for more.

Here's What to Look for in an Initial Flirtext from Your Crush:

1. Expect his first flirtext within 24–48 hours of giving him your number.

2. He will attempt to re-establish the connection you made in person by bringing up a conversation or something that happened when you met.

3. He will try to feel out what your schedule is to know when you're free to go out.

"I love Flirtexting because you can gauge a girl's intelligence. Can she spell? Is she witty? Does she know correct grammar?"

—Brett

GUYS' TEXTING SECRETS, TRUTHS, & CONFESSIONS REVEALED!

"Oldest trick in the book: The fake Mass Text. Make a text appear as if it's for everyone—but only send it to the girl you like. 'So who's out tonight?'. . . If she responds—you're in!" —Rich

"The best part about new phones is that they save your entire texting thread. This is extra awesome for us because we can look back through old conversations to bring up something specific a girl once said which makes us look like we were actually paying attention." —Luke

"I get a lot of texts from girls around 1 PM on Sunday's. My theory is they had a bad date last night, spent the morning brooding about it, and have resolved to start fresh by reconnecting with a 'good guy' from their past. Girls, I'm onto you." —John

"It's not all about getting laid . . . guys like the witty banter, constant real-time attention, teasing aspect as well!!" —Brett

Guy's Texting Turn-Offs

- "Sharing my texts with others without asking." —Chris

- "Unsolicited sexting." —Tyler

- "Using what you think is 'hip, cool' lingo, but really it just comes off as awkward, unnatural and trying too hard (i.e. 'You rockin n rollin tonight?'). You sound like my aunt." —Anthony

- "One letter responses." —Alex

- "Too much small talk." —Brett

- "Long-winded texts that go nowhere. 160 characters or less . . . preferably less." —Justin

Guy's Texting Turn Ons

- "Spontaneous, short and sweet, sexy texting." —Chris.

- "Phone calls are a turn on." —Rich

- "Playing hard to get. But not too hard. Then it just gets annoying." —Jake

- "Anything in list format helps. Guys tend to have ADD." —Brett

- "Just being honest and yourself. Lines don't work. Wit does." —Jeremy

Flirtextiquette

If you're flirting with the idea of flirtexting or are already a serial flirtexter, we urge you to mind your *ps* and *qs* and read up on the dos and don'ts of flirtexting. Practicing proper text etiquette, or *flirtextiquette*, will ensure a successful run of flirtexts. Flirtextiquette is a set of manners that will impress when used. We urge you to read up, manner up, and then text up.

Do Text:

1. *At the beginning of a relationship* to get to know him through flirty, witty banter.

2. *Light date* invites for a movie/drinks.

3. *Changing date* arrangements; i.e., time/place or when you're running late.

4. *Post-date* courtesy text.

5. *When you're thinking* about him and want him to know it.

6. *When you want to make him laugh.*

7. *When you want to catch-up* with an old fling but don't want to have a conversation over the phone.

8. *When he's calling* you and you don't like him, but feel the need to respond by making little effort.

9. *When you want to tell him* something that you're too shy to say in person.

10. *When you're long distance and texting* makes you feel closer while keeping your minutes down.

Don't Text:

1. *While on a date, in front of your date.*
   You may check your messages and quickly respond while you are on a bathroom break or if he gets up from the table.

2. *When it's really important.*
   Certain things should be said in person. Like: I want to break-up, I love you, Will you marry me? I'm pregnant, etc. It's insensitive and shows a lack of respect to belittle such important topics to a text message.

3. *When you're angry.*

   Text is not the time or place to start a heated conversation. If you must, send a pre-phone call text like: "Hey. Call me when you can. Need to chat." This lets him know something's up.

4. *When it's 3 AM and you're drunk.*

   We know it's tempting, but trust us—it's no fun waking up to a slew of embarrassing texts.

5. *RIGHT after fooling around.*

   Pillow-talk time is not the time to be checking your cell. It shows lack of interest and will make anyone lying next to you begin to feel self-conscious.

The Rule for Canceling a Date Over Text

Rule of thumb is to cancel the same way he asked you out. If he called to ask you out, then the right thing to do is to call back to cancel. If you send a text instead, then you're giving him signs that you are not that into him.

If he asked you out over text, then it's absolutely appropriate to text to cancel. Just keep in mind that date arrangements made over text are more likely to be canceled than if they were made by phone.

Post-Date Courtesy Text

Back in the day, Lady Mary from *Downton Abbey* would handwrite thank you notes to her potential suitors for taking her out. Today, she'd send a text. Any time a guy pays for your outing experience and you're still in the courting stages, it's common courtesy for you to send a thank you post-date text. The post-date courtesy text is thoughtful and short, not to mention the least us girls can do. He did just pay for your all-you-can-eat meal and that made-to-order mojito you had the bartender whip you up. A simple "thanks for such a yummy dinner had a great time stud!" will reinforce that you're a polite girl (whom he can bring home to Mom) and will lay down the groundwork for him to ask you out again.

> **Marathon Texting:** **Non-stop, all day flirtexting with a crush.**

More Texting No-Nos

"It's a turn-off when girls get angry at you for not engaging in a full texting conversation. If I'm out at dinner, I can't really text back and forth. I try to explain that, but people are very sensitive!" —Sebastian

While times exist where non-stop texting with a guy generates butterflies and excitement through much of your lackluster day, don't expect the following day to deliver the same. Guys tend to get burnt out from texting quicker

Rain Check Requests = Not That Interested

It's the oldest trick in the book. We agree to a date at first because we have nothing else to do Wednesday night. But when Wednesday afternoon rolls around, we decide we'd rather take a nap than get drinks with Matt.

So we send a text saying that we are terribly sorry, but something came up (i.e., you're feeling sick, your friend just broke up with her BF, your cat ODed on your Ambien, whatever) and we ask if we can have a "rain check." The truth is, if we really liked Matt then we would have been planning our outfit the night before and getting a manicure the day of.

Attention, ladies!! The same applies when he texts asking you for a "rain check." Our money is on the fact that that check will never be cashed. "Rain check" is a polite way of saying "I'm just not that into you." If he was interested and needed to reschedule he would have called. A text in this case is a cop-out.

Beware if he ever texts you, "rain check," take note and begin exploring other options. It's not you, honey, it's him.

than girls do. If a guy has a hectic morning of e-mails and phone calls, he'll tend to put the phone away for the afternoon to recoup, even if he really likes you.

You can generally sense a person's interest in you by their willingness to partake in a flirtexting marathon. For instance, if you text a guy first and he merely responds with a brief, non-flirty text when he normally gives you more, know to stop texting him and wait for him to respond later. Commonly, a guy who's interested in marathon texting will most likely text you first and throw out something extremely flirty and well thought-out. Proper etiquette with marathon-texts: Let the guy lead and always try to end it first.

Overloading Your Texts with Redundant Questions

Texting should be kept light and fun. Sending questions like: "What was it like growing up in Chicago?" or "What happened last night that you couldn't talk

texting tip

Text a Guy to the "Friend-Zone"

Just not that into him? Be clear but polite when placing guys in the friend zone.

Just throw in a pal, sport, kid, buddy, champ, or dude into any of your texts to him and he'll surely know where he stands. Example: "Hey Pal, dinner sounds fun but I'll need a rain check!"

Degree(s) of Interest

If you just had the best date of your life—we're talking can't-stop-smiling-you-lost-five-pounds-from-all-the-excitement date—then it's BEST to give him a call the next day to say thank you. If you really had that much fun, then we're sure he did too and would appreciate the call/confirmation. However, if your date was nice but nothing to write home about, then a sweet thank you text will suffice the following day. If the date is a complete flop and you hope he moves to Istanbul next week, your manners still shouldn't get in the way of your feelings. Texting, "Thank you again for dinner. Speak soon." the following day will let him know where he stands.

texting tip

about?" are no-nos. Might as well pin the kid down and shine a flashlight into his eyes. Don't ask things that will take up too much time and space to answer.

Feelings + Text = Bad Idea

It's hard to convey tone over text. It's safe to say that the tone in the majority of text exchanges is light and sarcastic. Therefore, writing things like, "I really don't see where this relationship is going" or "Who was that girl you were with last night?" don't hold as much

Don't Be That Girl.

We have noticed that some of our more popular girlfriends have become addicted and attached to their cell phones, in an unattractive way. Whether they are texting, BBMing, or e-mailing, their cells are always in their hand and they're always typing away on them. Don't be that girl. There is nothing more annoying than trying to hang out with someone who is constantly directing her attention toward other friends wirelessly. That's being social by being antisocial. And don't even get us started on the irritating sound consistent tapping away on the keyboard makes while we stare at your forehead. It's a surefire way to turn any guy off.

validity when said over text. Proper flirtextiquette is to not load your flirtexts with heavy statements and/ or questions about your feelings. It's best and more respectful to discuss these matters in person or over the phone. If you already have trouble with anxiety, we strongly discourage you from discussing feelings and important issues over text. Waiting for a response text can be an intense, emotionally driven situation. Sometimes you might find yourself saying outlandish things just to get a quicker reaction out of him. Be patient, Jane!

If You *Don't* Want a Date, Abbreviate

Listen up: the overuse of abbreviations, acronyms, and smilies in your flirtexts will put you on the next bus back to Single-town. If you want to avoid this be weary of how you write out your words and avoid sounding like you just stepped off the set of *Clueless*. While shortening words and letters is cute and funny when exchanged among your girlfriends, please don't use "brill" and "perf" in your flirtexts. They make you sound flighty. Constant abbreviations are totally girly and will make any guy roll his eyes—not laugh.

Obviously, you'll have to abbreviate some words in order to make your whole flirtext fit into one message. But sending "gr8 2 see u 2nite!" is not okay. If you need to cut down a few words so that it fits into one text, start by shortening words like "you" and "are" to "u" and "r." Catch our drift? If it still doesn't fit into one message, than turn that message into two texts, which is an appropriate solution.

The same goes for *overuse* of your symbols. Because we can't always tell tone over text, symbols can help create emphasis by letting the other person know we were only kidding. However, overuse of these makes you seem like an overzealous and hyper pre-teen girl on her way to a Justin Bieber concert. Let's reflect on these a moment:

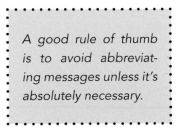

A good rule of thumb is to avoid abbreviating messages unless it's absolutely necessary.

:) —Okay, we know you think these guys are cute, but in reality they are unoriginal and a turn-off when over-used. Use sparingly, and only when you need it.

Hahas and LOLs—We really like these and think they are cute ways of signaling to your crush's ego that he is, in fact, making you laugh. It's also a good sign when he sends you one, because he thinks you're funny. These laughing signals however tend to be abused in flirtexts. Just know that every semi-funny line he sends doesn't warrant a laugh from you. Stay true, be genuine, and pick and choose your LOLs. After all, he is going to be sending you all sorts of funny texts to try to impress. Don't make it too easy for him.

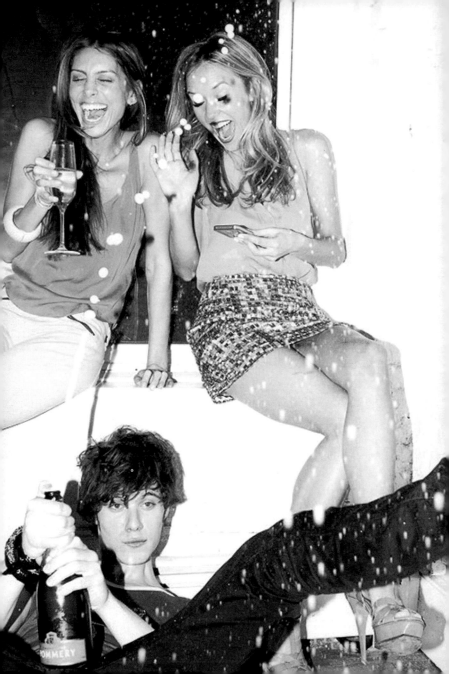

PART TWO:

game on

"It's okay to put yourself out
there in a text. Telling me you miss me
or want to see me is not a sign of weakness."

—Rich

CONFIDENCE: YOU CAN'T FAKE IT

Confidence plays a major role in helping any woman land a great guy. It's the one characteristic that sets you apart from the rest of the pack and attracts men like magnets. Confidence is a trait that you can't fake, no matter how hard you play "the game" or how good of a flirt you are. We have no doubt that with confidence on your side, you will always end up on top (pun intended).

Confident women are sure of themselves inside and out. Everything about them exudes certainty and assurance. They are usually fearless and always go after what they want. They know their weaknesses just as well as they know their strong points. They're able to laugh at themselves and aren't afraid of putting themselves out there. They'd rather be up-front and take chances than not try at all.

> *There is something about a self-assured, intelligent, quick-witted girl who knows where she's heading in life that'll always turn heads.*

Being a confident person shows in everything you do. It's in the way you walk, talk, and guess what, it's in the way you flirtext. Therefore, when you text, mean what you say. Stand by your ideals and values. Don't change your views for the sake of thinking someone else will appreciate them. Be proud of who you are, where you're from, and what you stand for. Having this awareness at all times, including when you flirtext, will benefit you tremendously.

You know how the saying goes: "When it rains, it pours." Ever wonder why the second you're off the

Dating the Flirtexting Way: Two people casually spending time together for the purpose of seeing if they want to eventually become exclusive. You are allowed to, and absolutely should, flirtext and date other people if you are not exclusive. The best thing you can do for yourself while single is to keep your options open. Once you have mutually decided to date exclusively (i.e., you only want to be flirtexting each other), then a talk will "seal the deal" for you to officially be boyfriend and girlfriend. (For rules on when flirtexting is considered cheating see Part Three.)

market you become flooded with attention from eligible suitors? That aura of confidence that you wear so well attracts guys like honeybees to clover. The secure feeling that comes with being in a relationship is what helps you let your guard down and allows you to be your natural self. This makes you more approachable. **The secret is exuding that same confidence in your flirtext.**

Think Like a Guy

The two of us have been told many times that we think like guys, which we realize is an abnormality of the conventional chemical make-up. When it comes to dating, men and women typically have very different attitudes. Guys tend to take a more laid-back and carefree approach, while ladies sometimes allow our emotional side to complicate things.

Let's start with the guys. If a girl they like likes them back, they're thrilled. If she doesn't, they move on. Guys don't over analyze the things we say, nor do they drive themselves crazy trying to figure out why we turned them down. Guys roll with the punches in order to avoid drama, and for the most part, aim to please. This attitude is very apparent in their straight-to-the point flirtexts. Example: "When can I see you?" or "Come over."

Girls, on the other hand, we're a bit more complex with our approach. We tend to let our feelings get in the way of rational thinking, or **text when we know we shouldn't.** We lay our cards out too quickly, displaying eagerness within our texts. We're so used to doing what we say we're going to do, **if he doesn't text when he says he will, he's a goner.** We discovered that by

Give him a taste of his own medicine and watch as your bases become fully loaded.

thinking like a guy, we avoid unwanted stress and anxiety in our relationships. Displaying that same laissez-faire attitude within your flirtext will impress the guy on the receiving end and make you more desirable.

Guys love women who are laid-back and easy-going. Having this attitude makes their lives easier, and makes being with you more enjoyable. Try to remember this the next time a potential boyfriend (a PBF) flirtexts you bad news. Say you got two fifth row tickets to a baseball game and invited your crush. You can't wait to impress him with your seats behind the dugout and your knowledge of random baseball trivia. A few hours before the game you get the following text from him, "Hey I'm sorry something came up at work and I cant make the game tonight. I'll call you later." **Strike one.**

Here's where displaying a laid-back attitude in your flirtext will benefit you. Even though you're upset he canceled, the trick is not to display your degree of disappointment in your response. Don't get emotional. Instead, think like a guy. Ask yourself how he would respond if the situation were reversed and you were the one canceling. Responding with, "No worries about the change-up. I'll just call in a replacement hitter," will impress your crush and show you're a cool girl who can roll with the punches. Or, if you're a bit more forward, "No worries! Although I was looking forward to going to first base. Next time ;)" Watch as

your nonchalant yet flirty response has him reschedul-
ing the next time your team has a home game.

Sporting a laid-back, easy-going 'tude will greatly
benefit you. Having this mind-set will become apparent
in your flirtexts and will help you land on the winning
side. *Now play ball!*

Hook a Guy with Your Text

We all operate by the saying we want what we can't
have. This has proven to be true in life, in business,
but especially so in love. Therefore, it's no secret: *guys
want what they can't have*. Here's how they rationalize: If a girl they are interested in proves to be an easy
catch (i.e., responds to all of his flirtexts immediately
and/or agrees to go on dates with him last minute)
then they eventually get turned off by her "too available" attitude and move on. No need to analyze this
because it's always the case. **Hooking a guy doesn't
have to be a game; it's common sense that can be
taught.**

Aware of men's short attention spans and competitive
edge in dating, we've incorporated the "want what you
can't have" style into our flirtexting method. We've
instituted this as a way to stand above the rest. By holding back your level of attraction at first, you're setting
yourself up as a challenge, making him more intrigued.
Then, as you begin to open up to him and grow closer,
your initial resistance will make him feel like he's earned
something by winning your attention. Compare this to a
young kid whom you let win a game of cards. The child
is so happy they won, they begin to like you even more.

texting tip

The Rules

Greg Behrendt of *He's Just Not That Into You*, and every guy we know say that if he's not calling you, he doesn't like you. By this logic, if he's not texting you, chances are he probably doesn't like you . . . (at least not in the way you like him).

To hook a guy in the beginning stages of dating, you need to give him a little taste of how cool and fun you are, but then play a little coy so you set yourself up as a challenge. *We call this a strategic tease.* Entice him by making your first text exchanges light, witty, and flirty, so he doesn't feel intimidated. Once he begins to respond quickly, you have him hooked and now it's time to pull back.

For example, when a guy sends you a random text, one that he thinks is funny, clever, and certainly worthy of a response, don't respond. You aren't required to respond to every text. Pick and choose your flirtexts. He'll begin to wonder if your non-response was due to him "turning you off" by something he wrote. Guys have admitted to us they rationalize dead air the same way we do (only for not as long). He's wondering if you didn't get his joke or if his text didn't go through. He's rationalizing all sorts of crap in order to keep his ego intact. By not giv-

texting tell-all

As a flirtexter, you learn not to tell a guy that you want to marry him and have all his babies from the get-go. You don't want to inflate his ego by letting him know how into him you are. Instead, you want to remain in the "I could take you or leave you because I have, like, a gazillion hot, amazing men in my life" category. In order to do this, we encourage playing a light game of hard to get.

Note: If you are one of those girls who think games are immature and pointless then pay extra special attention. When played responsibly, strategic games are actually very helpful and produce results. Girls who seem too eager and easy to please turn guys off. Know the right amount of game playing is necessary to reel him in..

ing him the response he wants or feels he deserves, he'll begin to want it—and you—that much more. If this has ever happened to you then you know exactly what it feels like. It's absolute torture until you get a response. We may play a few harmless games now and again, but we're not one to torture a man's soul. So when he texts again, (the ones that like you always will) respond away.

If you think for some reason, "Well, what if he doesn't know I like him" and find the need to keep in constant touch as a means of assuring your undeniable *like* for him, then know you're blazing the wrong path, sister. Guys don't easily stray if they really like a girl. Stay true to yourself and be a little patient. By not responding to his every text and taking your time to write back, he'll begin to want you more. After all, good things come to those who wait.

Another easy way to hook a guy with your flirtexts is instead of responding to his jokes with a typical "LOL," hit him back with an equally witty, (if not better), comeback. Guys are so used to girls feeding their egos by telling them how funny they are or laughing at their not-so-funny jokes. No ma'am, not us. Our money's on the fact that he's probably texted this joke or one like it to a different girl at a different time. Therefore responding with a "Lol u r so funny" is predictable and expected. Instead try responding in a way that will set you apart from the rest and keep him on his toes: "What's this nonsense about a chicken crossing the road?"

Teach Him How to Treat You

"It's pretty simple. If you text a girl late night and she writes you back, doesn't matter what she says, she wants to hook up." —Jason

Guys like rules. Really, they'd be thrilled to have a road map describing exactly what to do in order to get the girl that they want. You set the standard by treating others as you would like to be treated. In the early stages of courtship, it is therefore imperative that you set up expectations early enough so that he knows how to behave and communicate with you. This sets the tone for your relationship thereafter.

> **PBF (Potential Boyfriend): A crush. You may have known him for two years or two minutes.**

You can easily teach a potential boyfriend (PBF) how to treat you through text messaging. Say, for example, you went on one or two dates with a new crush. Then, one night around 1 AM, you get the following LNBT (late night booty text), "hey . . . what are you doooin?" You have three options: You can respond right away. You can respond in the morning, during "daylight" hours. Or, you can not respond at all. If you choose to respond that night, (we're not mad at ya) just beware that you could be setting yourself up to be placed in his "LNBT" category, and most likely continue to only receive texts late at night from this particular suitor. Your second option is to respond the next day with a message letting him know you're still interested, just not at 1 AM! If he truly likes you, he'll get the picture and call or text during more appropriate hours from here on out. If you choose to not respond at all, don't feel guilty. After all, it's 1 AM and you just started dating. What does he expect? And, may we add, what kind of girl does he think you are?!

All we ask is that you think about this next time a crush reaches out to you late at night. Do you want to be the girl that he makes plans to see in advance and takes on fun dates, or the girl he knows he can see late night without any notice or effort on his part?

If you want the former, then set the standard from the beginning. If he truly likes you, he'll chill with the LNBT and contact you during non-booty text hours.

LNBT (Late Night Booty Text): Any text sent from a crush past 11 p.m. with an invite to meet up.

"If I'm having multiple text convos,
which I usually am, when a girl says
something clever, funny, or anything sweet,
I'll just cut, copy, and paste it to
the next conversation."

—Richard

CREATING THE
BEST POSSIBLE TEXT

There are some things in life that should be avoided and awkward phone conversations are one of them. For everything else, there's texting. Most guys feel talking over the phone puts them on the spot to constantly entertain with funny jokes and tantalizing stories. Take this example:

Jenna: Hello?

Ben: Hey, Jenna. This is Ben.

Jenna: Who?

Ben: Ben. We met the other night at the bar.

Jenna: Oh yeah, hey. What's going on?

Ben: Oh, not much. So, how's your foot?

Jenna: Excuse me?

Ben: Remember? You got stepped on while we were dancing. We almost got into a fight with the girl who did it.

Jenna: Oh yeah, (awkward laugh) I forgot about that. Yeah, it's fine. A little bruised, but I'll live.

Ben: Oh good. Thought they might have to amputate. (dead air)

Jenna: (another forced laugh)

Ben: Uh, just wanted to call to say I, umm, I wanted to see what you're up to later tonight or this week. I was, uh, thinking we, you know could maybe catch a flick or grab some dinner . . . (long pause) if you were free, ya know? (clearing throat)

Jenna: Oh, cool. Yeah, let me look at my calendar and call you back.

Later . . . no call back

If you ask a guy how he feels about phone calls, we'll bet he says he *hates* talking on the phone. Guys *love* to text because they feel less pressure than when calling. Say goodbye to blurting out dumb phrases and pointless stories all for the sake of avoiding awkward silence. For all these reasons, guys love to text, so girls MUST learn how to flirtext.

The following is what that same awkward phone convo between Ben and Jenna would sound like via flirtext:

Ben: Jenna, you've got dance moves that would put Paula Abdul out of work. How's that crushed foot of yours today?

> *One of the biggest advantages texting has to offer is complete control over what you say.*

Jenna: Hey! I did outdo Paula, huh? The foot's a little bruised, but nothing some ice and a cold drink won't fix!

Recipe for Success

1. Know what you want.

2. Determine your Best Possible Text.

3. Know when to press send.

Ben: How about I'll get you that drink if you promise not to dance too close to me and make me feel bad about my dancing skills?

Jenna: Deal. But I can't make any promises about the dancing. You saw me last night—I'm a machine ;)

The first part of successful flirtexting begins with creating the Best Possible Text (BPT).

BPT (Best Possible Text): A text that says exactly what you want and in the best possible way. In order to create this, your message has to be strategically planned and aimed at getting your desired response.

You can tell a LOT about a person by what they text, making it a necessity to always put your best text forward. As quick as we are to put our best foot forward when meeting someone new, we must remember to do the same with our texts.

> *You always want your flirtext to include just the right amount of humor, mystery, and sass to make you seem desirable and to leave your crush wanting more.*

Putting the right ingredients into your flirtext will show him you're interested, and keep his interest piqued. Luckily, text allows you the time to compose this perfect potion!

A valuable lesson we've learned in life is to try and take a step back and think about what we're doing and what we want at any given moment. Taking two seconds to consciously think about our actions before doing them can help reduce mistakes and curb our impulsive nature. For example, if you're at dinner and the waiter sets a huge plate of fries in front of you, taking a second to recognize if you actually want those fries before impulsively reaching for them can make all the difference. The same goes for texting.

How to Create the Best Possible Text (BPT)

1. *Know what you want:*

   Figure out what you want so you can strategically craft a text to get your desired response. Do you want him to ask you out? Be your boyfriend? Call? Once you know this the rest is easy.

2. *Forecast obstacles:*

   Think about all the things that could possibly get in your way of getting what you desire. Try to remember if he said anything about his weekend plans when you spoke to him earlier. Is he going out of town? Is it his best friend's birthday? It's always a good idea to have a little 411 on your honey's weekly activities before hitting him up. You wouldn't want to ask him to do something when you can mathematically prove he will turn you down. This step will ensure your attempt won't be wasted.

3. *Brainstorm BPTs:*

Now that you know what you want and can't predict any obstacles getting in your way, create a BPT, a sub-tle and strategic text message to get what you want. You must never write the first thing that comes to mind. If you draw a blank or have doubts about what to write, ask a friend. If that doesn't help, pick up our book for example texts, or go to our Flirtexting Facebook page and send us a message or send us a tweet @flirtexting. Do whatever it is that you need to do in order to feel you have narrowed it down to the absolute BPT.

4. *Ask a friend:*

It's always a good idea to get a second opinion when creating BPTs. It's difficult being flirty, sassy, funny, and impeccably dressed 100% of the time. At times when you're not on top of your game and need a clever flirtext, friends are your best resource. They can help turn your run-of-the-mill text into a BPT. Since they are not emotionally involved like you are, their ideas are usually more playful. Best part: you get all the credit! Take into consideration that what you may think is a sweet, lighthearted mes-sage may read as "trying too hard" to someone else. Your best friend can help you maneuver this situation—after all, that's what they're there for.

5. *Leave an opt out:*

A Rules Girl always leaves her options open. In cases when you're asking to make plans with a guy, if possible, try and create an "opt out" in your text in case he comes up with something better or is unable to make it. Meaning, don't ever commit to something before he agrees to it first. For example, never text, "I'm going to the movies on Friday night, do you want to go?" That statement is too definite. If you want to see him, movie or not, then instead text, "Thinking about catching a movie Friday night. Interested?" This leaves your plans more open-ended, giving him the opportunity to suggest something better.

Knowing When to Press Send

"Because it helps me distinguish the desperate from the not desperate girls. Response time says a lot about a person." —Josh

You just received a flirtext from your crush. You're stoked because you've been thinking about him all day and were wondering if he was doing the same. The minute you receive his text you begin writing the first thing that comes to mind, and then press send. Five, ten, thirty minutes go by and he still hasn't written back. You begin to

FLIP out and are certain his silence is due to your lame, impulsive text.

In the quiet meantime, you start driving yourself crazy coming up with a half dozen better flirtexts which you're certain would have elicited a faster response. You swear to yourself that when and if he finally writes back, you'll be more patient with your next response to ensure the "haha" you so rightfully deserve. Or, at the very least, a timely response.

Now that you've gotten your message in place, the second part of successful flirtexting is knowing when to press send. Unfortunately, part of being a girl means getting overly excited about a simple text from a crush. A text can escalate that already neurotic butterflies-in-stomach feeling, and drive the common

....

BPT thought process . . .

You want to see a movie with him tonight and you can't recall anything important he'd be doing since you talked to him yesterday, and he didn't mention anything. You know he's a Vince Vaughn fan and it just so happens Vaughn's new movie is premiering this weekend. You create a text that's enticing enough to ensure a "yes" or at the very least a date in the near future.

It reads: "Any interest in seeing the new Vince Vaughn movie? Rule #76: No excuses. Play like a champion." *(Wedding Crashers)*

....

Don't let the girly-girl in you get in the way of your game and control. If he texts you, then the ball is in your court and you hold the power. We recommend holding onto that power for as long as your manicured hands can.

sense right out of a girl! In other words, upon receiving his text, you feel the need to respond instantly, 'cause let's face it, you l-o-v-e him. This a bad idea.

Just because it's speedy technology does not mean you need to be instant with your response! The first text you think of is probably impulsive and driven by emotion. The trick is to tone down any excitement you may have and resist the urge to write the first thing that pops into your head. There certainly is no rush when it comes to flirtexting.

Unlike phone calls or F2F conversations, where you are put on the spot to be clever and witty, *text gives you the power of time*. The secret lies in the way you use this time. By having the element of time on your side in flirtexting, you hold the power and upper hand. Yes, it's as simple as that.

Admit it. In the back of every flirtexter's mind there's an unspoken timeline pertaining to when one texts and when one responds. It's all really a game of catch-me-if-you-can. Responding at just the right moment is key when trying to land a man via text. If you respond too quickly you could come across looking desperate. Wait too long and you might come off looking uninterested. Knowing *when* to press send is just as important as what you are sending … if not more so. Allow us to explain.

While the phone call and F2F conversation is more instant, text allows you to determine your speed according to your desire. You can respond to text messages *instantly,* exuding interest and eagerness; *delay your response,* conveying a sense of mystery and that you're hard-to-get; or ultimately *not respond at all,* which can mean one of two things: you're not interested in him *or* you're not interested in his flirtext. Use time to adjust your game to your needs. Whether you want to be straight and to the point or a coquette, the ball is in your court. Use it to your advantage.

The same way *The Rules* told us to wait a day or two before returning his phone call, we're telling you to keep this same state of mind—hold off a bit—when responding to his text. This signals you're not an easy catch. Wait until something brilliant and witty comes to you even if it means responding the following day.

Waiting It Out: Every flirtexting situation differs, in which case the response time will vary. However, the longest you should hold out when responding back to his flirtext is twenty-four hours. Anything beyond that reads as uninterested.

Delaying your response works to your advantage the same way his delayed response works for you. When you pause your response, your potential boyfriend may start second guessing his text, as well as his approach. While you're composing something clever, or getting on with your life, he's going crazy wondering if you still like him. **Guys have revealed to us that they go nuts waiting for our response just like we do.** He may not admit it or show any signs, but he's freaking out a little. Guys are just better at keeping their emotions hidden, while girls wear our hearts on our sleeves. They hide it, we analyze it. We're different creatures. If he admitted that it drove him crazy waiting for your response he would lose a little game and a whole lot of manhood. So when you come back with the perfect response, he'll be quietly thrilled, which you'll see firsthand when he responds back right away. Trust that by not responding instantly you'll reap the benefits in the long run.

The delayed text works best in the most critical of situations. Whether you're head-over-heels or just interested in getting to know him better, the best thing you can do is hold back your response a bit.

We KNOW that holding back your response is hard to do. But may we remind you, it's not like he showed up on your doorstep with a dozen roses and a cupcake. It's a text.

Yes, texting back immediately leaves you with that instant gratification you so desperately need. But remember, this feeling is followed by a slow fall into depression when you don't hear back immediately. It's like a sugar high you don't want to be on. What you want to do is feed his ego and make him feel like he's the luckiest guy in the world when you finally write back.

> *Text gives you the advantage of time and therefore the power.*

This technique is probably similar

Stop!

Do not respond immediately to any text, even if you think you have the perfect response. Call your BFF, watch something on Netflix, go on a run ... whatever! Do anything to distract yourself. Remember, he's lucky to be getting a flirtext from you. Make him realize it by making him wait. Always leave him wanting more.

texting tip

to the strategy you used to get his attention in the first place. You most likely flirted with someone else in his direct eyesight to make him notice you. Finally, after making him sweat the whole night, you gave *him* your number. This gave him the ultimate satisfaction because, in a sense, he's won. (Not that it was a game or anything.)

Here we list different timelines for texting scenarios and what it means by how long we take to respond. These approximate timelines pertain to budding relationships and do not apply if you are texting back a friend or family member. And it doesn't count if you're in a serious relationship. We advise using these in the initial six weeks of dating.

Waiting it out means he's sweating it out.

Texting Timelines

1. His text—"What are u doing tonight"—at 5:30 PM

Your type	When you respond	What it means about you
Jane	5:32 PM	You love him and now he knows it and has all the power. Don't do this.
The Romantic	6:00 PM	You like him a lot. You want to see him and don't care if he knows it.
The Chill Girl	7:30 PM	You think you like him but don't really know yet. Perhaps you'll know more based on his response.
The Bad Ass	8:30 PM	You like him but want to field your options. He's not the only one to ask you out tonight. He better have a good plan to keep your interest.
The Shameless	1:30 AM to 5 AM	Oh, sweetie (We know what you're up to. And we still love you.)

| The Busy Girl | 3:00 PM the next day | By taking this long to respond you probably had a lot going on. You're giving off a catch-me-if-you-can 'tude. |

2. *His text—"What's going on?"—2 PM after two weeks of silence.*

Your type	When you respond	What it means about you
Jane	2:15 PM	Who are we kidding? You're so happy he texted you completely forgot it's been two whole weeks!
The Romantic	3:00 PM	You kept a positive outlook and promised yourself if it's meant to be, he'll reach out. You write back in hopes of seeing him very soon.
The Chill Girl	5:00 PM	You're psyched that he's back but are in no rush to let him know it.

The Badass	The following day	You give him a little taste of his own medicine and don't make it easy for him to get ahold of you quickly.
The Busy Girl	Won't respond till his second attempt for contact	He's been out of contact for two weeks. WTF! Obvy he's interested in you because he's re-establishing contact. But just because he's back doesn't mean you're going to respond right away. Therefore, you wait until he texts again to earn your attention a bit more.

texting tell-all

Plan B?

If a guy texts you to ask you out to dinner a few hours before the reservation, keep in mind his plans may have fallen through which means you're plan B. When a guy really likes you and wants to take you out to dinner, he asks a few days in advance like a gentleman.

The Waiting Game

"The anticipation of the response is exciting to me. There's a moment of wow . . . did that just cross the line? And then she texts back and the mild anxiety turns to adrenaline and you feel like you're a pimp again."—Gene

It's Saturday afternoon. You and your PBF were texting back and forth earlier that day about insignificant nothings. Now it's 3 PM and you want to know if you are going to see him tonight. (After all, you're not about to waste a new going-out top if he's not going to see it.) You decide to text him: "Big plans tonight?"

Ideally, he responds within thirty minutes with "you tell me ;)." But he doesn't, so you wait. And wait. You go to the gym for a spin class and hope no one sees that your phone is in the cup holder. Lame. Class is over and still silence. You head over to get some caffeine, because at this rate it's looking like a long night. While enjoying your coffee your phone buzzes and as you lunge into your bag to grab it you burn your hand. UGH! It's only your BFF asking what you're wearing tonight. Finally, you hop into the shower and decide if he doesn't write back by the time you're out, it's his loss and you're moving on. Then to spite him, you decide you're going to wear that new top anyways because you're on the prowl to replace "Mr.–I'm–too–busy–to–text–back." Whatever.

It's Just a Text

Here's the thing: Guys in general are naturally more nonchalant about responding in a timely manner than girls. When he's at the gym, he's at the gym. When he's eating lunch, he's eating lunch. He might read your text immediately, but he won't respond until it's appropriate to do so (i.e., after the gym or after lunch). Guys don't freak out when they receive a text, read it to everyone around them, and ask their friends to help create the best possible text.

This time lapse may appear like he's playing games or not that into you, when in reality, it's just him being a dude. Try to train yourself to think differently about why he hasn't responded. Know that his non-response has nothing to do with you and everything to do with him (unless, of course, you sent a lame text). **Whatever you do, please don't send him another text just for the sake of getting**

texting tip

Did You Get My Text?

Be wary of guys who use excuses, "I lost my phone" or "my phone died." We've all used these before and know they're lies, lies, lies. He got your message and just didn't respond. Therefore, refrain from asking "did you get my text?" because it's a lost cause and you'll come off looking like Jane if you do.

him to respond. Guys deem that desperate and it's a huge turn off. Put it this way: Jane would send another text and then one to his friend trying to find her guy. Don't be Jane.

Try not to let the time lapse get to you because let's face it, we know what happens to you when it does. He'll have you second guessing your text and re-reading it a million times. Thoughts begin racing: *Was it something I said? Did he not get my joke? Did his battery die??* Not only are these frantic theories a huge waste of time, but they're all pathetic excuses we come up with to make ourselves feel better.

The act of texting is casual. Therefore, taking a little time to respond back is permitted and even admired. Try to remember this while you're waiting for his response. Even if you're secretly going crazy inside, the key is to create a laid-back attitude about the situation, much like our male counterparts do. Set the phone aside and go on with your day/life. You are a chill girl who has better things to do than wait around in agony for a text response. We guarantee he will respond when he can.

Realizing you hold all the power in that little cell of yours is key to a long road of successful flirtexting. A well-worded message sent at the time you desire can help navigate the direction you want your relationship to go. **Remember, what you send is just as important as when you send it, and the time you take in responding says a lot about your level of interest.** Alert: Your popularity may improve by using this formula. Don't be surprised if your inbox is full by the time you're done reading. And no, we won't pay your next phone bill.

Subtext: What We Mean vs What We Text

Texting can leave a lot up to misinterpretation. It's important that flirtexters understand how to read the subtext of a text. **The subtext of a text is what we really mean by what we text.** Below are some common text messages guys and girls send to each other, and what they really mean.

His Text	His Subtext
You out tonight?	Are you out drinking? If so I want to hook up with you.
I think I'm staying home later. Let me know if you want to meet up.	I'm too lazy to get out of bed but if you're drunk and horny and want to make out later, I'd get out of bed to let you in for that.
We should hang sometime.	We should hang sometime.
I have to cancel tonight I have a work thing.	I upgraded my plans to something better that may include another girl or hanging with my buddies.

Going out with the guys tonight.	You should make other plans.
I've been meaning to call you! How's life?	I thought if I called you'd think I liked you more than I actually do, which is why I'm texting you.
I'm sorry I fell asleep.	I didn't want to wait for you so I decided to masturbate and call it a night.
I'm not sure what my plans are later.	I'm keeping my options open because I sense something big may come through in a bit.

Her Text	Her Subtext
Sorry I never responded to your text Friday night. I lost my phone and just got it back!	I don't like you, but I feel bad ignoring you so I'll pretend I lost my phone to be nice.
Hi there. So great meeting you last night as well.	I was wasted when I gave you my number. Who is this?
Did you try to call?	Please call.
What are you doing?	Pay attention to me.

I'd love to go out with you but I have a boy-friend.	I'm going to pretend to have a boyfriend so you stop asking me out.
I'm so busy with work this week. I'll text you next week when things slow down.	Don't wait by the phone. I'm not busy at all, I just don't like you.
Are you going to Matt's party tonight?	Please come to Matt's party tonight. I just got my nails done and I'm wearing a new dress just for you.
I like you a lot but I'm not looking for a rela-tionship.	I'm just not that into you. If I were, I wouldn't be ending things over a text.

Texting Under the Influence (TUI)

Drunk texts are the pink elephants of our night owl existence. As much as you would like to deny and for-get the fact that you drunk-texted, you can't. Honey, that crap is cemented into your phone! The only thing worse than waking up to discover your text log full of outgoing flirtexts that you don't remember sending, is reading those texts. They were most likely sent to a current crush or an old flame suggesting things you never would have suggested while sober. Not to men-tion they are probably filled with multiple misspellings

texting tell-all

"We all do it and live to tell the story the next day. It's the strangest thing. No matter who I'm out with, someone, after a few cocktails, always thinks it's the most brilliant idea to text something to their current crush or old flame. It's like an episode of *Sex and the City*. I've seen all forms of prevention for the drunk text: handing over your phone to a friend, signing up for a service that prevents you from dialing your crush's number past 10 PM, making your friend swear not to let you dial anyone but your mom. The reality of all this is grim and short-lived. As you down cocktail number three, the chances of your not texting your crush are about as slim as Samantha vowing to become celibate. We all break after some point and think Carrie Bradshaw couldn't have written a better text herself." —Olivia

and incomplete sentences, making you look ridiculous. You are so embarrassed by these texts that you turn your lights off and go back to bed, hoping that when you wake up for the second time it was all a bad dream. At first you may not believe it, but trust us, we'll explain how there's life after a night of Texting Under the Influence . . . or TUI.

The TUI phenomenon happens because alcohol lowers our inhibitions and impairs our rational thinking, making us more likely to say exactly how we feel without censoring ourselves like we normally would. And being that text messaging is instant and easy, it's our go-to when that boost of liquid courage gets ahold of us, making TUI all too common.

> **T.U.I. (texting under the influence):** Texting under the influence of any mood altering substance such as drugs, alcohol, a great Ryan Gosling movie, etc.

If you drink alcohol while in the presence of your cell phone, then sooner or later you are going to want to drunk text. It's human nature. We too have been guilty of TUI a time or two and know the effect alcohol has on our inhibitions. That is why we strongly recommend never, *ever* doing it. In this chapter we include some explanations behind common drunk texting scenarios and a few sweet tips on how to avoid TUI all together. And let's not forget the guys, also guilty as charged. In addition to helping you save face, we've also included suggestions on how to handle their late night texts and inappropriate booty calls.

Scenario 1: "I look ridiculously good tonight."
You just had your eyebrows waxed, your hair looks the best it has all month, and your new DVF number is earning compliments all around. You're out with your friends, and think what a great idea it would be to text

a crush (whom you haven't heard from in a while) to see what he's doing tonight. He's still on your mind and you think that tonight's the perfect opportunity to see him because, well, you look hot! The alcohol has given you just enough courage to get your phone out and begin to compose a drunken text to the unsuspecting lad.

Truth: Step away from the phone, Miss von Furstenberg! Yes, you look hot. But hey, guess what? Your crush can't see that. Word to the wise: Texting late at night while under the influence is never the right time to be catching up with an old crush. Plus, with your late night text, you've pretty much agreed to make out with him without him having to lift a finger.

Furthermore, your texting him after hours is a sign that you are swinging solo, sister. Basically, due to this needy reach out, you've set the tone for the type of relationship you are willing to have.

How to Avoid Scenario 1: Remind yourself that you're out for a reason. You're drinking to let loose, have fun with your friends, and forget about the stresses of school, work, and the crises of your personal life (including long-lost BFs). Distract yourself from your phone. Go find a guy at the bar and make funny conversation to keep yourself entertained. This is a great way to get whoever else is on your mind off of it. A good laugh is always better than a cry of humiliation in the morning.

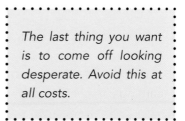
The last thing you want is to come off looking desperate. Avoid this at all costs.

Or

If you're really hung up on getting in touch with him, make a pact with yourself. Tell yourself that you will call or text him tomorrow during daylight hours. Planning something like a phone call to a crush can be exciting, plus when it's done appropriately—aka not in a desperate, drunken stupor—he will be genuinely pleased and impressed. Additionally, this will a) give you time to see if you still want to text/call him tomorrow when you're sober (the true test) and b) prevent him from losing any interest in you because you texted him while inebriated.

Scenario 2: Can't let go of the past and move on.
You just ran into your ex-boyfriend's brother at the hotspot where you and your FBF (favorite boyfriend) first met. All of a sudden, the DJ spins your favorite Coldplay song on his turntable. You begin to get sentimental

texting tip

Texting Sponsor: Friends Don't Let Friends T.U.I.!

Need a reminder to text your sponsor? Go to www.Flirtexting.com, pick up a set of "Texting Sponsor" friendship bracelets, and never send another T.U.I again.

because that was "your song" with him. As fate would have it, at that very moment you see a guy who looks just like your ex walk by. Your heart skips a beat as you pick up your phone to drop him a line about the crazy coincidences that just occurred.

Truth: In this scenario, you either just broke up with someone or never received closure on a very significant relationship. You can't fathom him being with anyone else. You dwell on your past times together, and the mere thought of seeing his name pop up in your inbox makes your knees go weak. Bottom line, you still have serious feelings for this guy. There are so many things left unsaid, and the alcohol, mixed with all the coincidences, has made you want to text him. You miss him.

How to Avoid Scenario 2: Friends don't let friends TUI. Appoint one of your best friends a "sponsor" that you always, we repeat: *always,* text whenever you feel the desire to contact this guy. Let this person know that whenever you get the desire to text him, you will text your sponsor instead. Texting your friend will serve as your safety net for doing something you would later regret. In return, she will most likely remind you of his bad qualities and make texting him less appealing.

The logic behind this is that your sponsor acts as a sponge, allowing you to release any of those "loving feelings" on her instead of him. By texting her first, you allow time to pass by when your desire to text him was the strongest. Hopefully by the time she writes you back your desire to text him is gone.

Alert Alert

Drunk texting an old flame puts you in a Danger Zone! Not only are you drunk, which makes you ten times more emotional, but 1:30 AM is not the time to be opening up about your feelings. In the end you will only be putting yourself and him through more pain. We know it's hard to remember this at a time when all signs point in his direction, but you're not in a relationship with him for good reason.

No matter how many good times you had together, it ended because one of your hearts wasn't in it. Therefore there's absolutely no point in dragging this out any longer if he's not your Mr. Right. We know this isn't the answer you want to hear because he's the one you hold a candle for. But sweetie, life goes on and you will rise again. We guarantee it.

Scenario 3: Late night invites for drinks, a date, or make-out sesh.

It's 1 AM and you get a late-night drunk text from a PBF that says, "Whath arer you dooing?" You could be out on the town celebrating a friend's birthday or sitting at home watching TV. Either way, you have mixed feelings about his text. You're flattered that he is thinking about you, but at the same time, a little pissed off because this is clearly a drunk text. You like him, but are not sure how to respond.

We've asked all of our guy friends about this and the answer is always the same: texts sent late night are purely sexual.

Like we said before, in life as well as in dating, it's your responsibility to teach someone how to treat you. If you entertain his texts and late night pleas, don't be surprised if you start seeing a pattern of LNBT from this guy. That is why you have to take control from the get-go.

How to Avoid Scenario 3: If you like this guy and see potential for a future relationship, then ignore his LNBT. By not responding, you let him know that you're rejecting his LNBT's, not him. If he likes you, he'll take the hint and contact you the next day, most likely to try and hang out earlier. Be sure to let him know that you got his message but aren't the kind of gal to give in so easily.

Scenario 4: You texted him late night and he's not texting you back.

You spoke to him earlier and know he is out on the town tonight. It's midnight now, and he said he would text you later to see what you are up to. You're having a good time partying with your friends and into your second drink begin thinking about him while incessantly checking your phone to see if he texted. When you absolutely can't stand it anymore, you text him even though you know you shouldn't, to see what he's doing and he doesn't text you back.

Truth: Even though we are engaged in a texting culture, guys' manners shouldn't disappear because it's easier to approach you. Nor should your morals and class give way to their easy plays.

Truth: This is a case of "actions speak louder than words," where his words weren't in line with his behavior. And ultimately, his actions or lack thereof, are what you should be concentrating on. So by contacting him anyway, you are setting yourself up for rejection if he turns you down. Take his silence as a sign showing you where you stand. Know when to graciously bow-out.

The UGLY Truth: If you text a guy late at night and he doesn't respond, he's most likely with another girl or doesn't want to see you. You can contemplate all you want about why he's not responding, but the truth is he didn't want to make out. After all, he is a guy, and texting him late night is basically like offering yourself up to him on a silver platter. If he didn't respond, and you know he wasn't sleeping, take the hint and move on! He clearly has.

How to Avoid Scenario 4: Try to leave your conversations open-ended, allowing either one of you to get in touch. Meaning instead of saying, "Text me later" say "Let's keep in touch." This helps to avoid this kind of miscommunication altogether. Therefore, if you do text him and he doesn't respond, you can walk away guilt free knowing you did your part.

texting tell-all

Always Double-Check

"I just got off the phone with my ex-boyfriend, Jeff, to tell him that I was moving to his city. I totally played it cool on the phone and alluded to the fact that it was no biggie and maybe I'd see him around sometime, when really I was jumping off the walls excited to be moving to the same city as him. Literally two seconds after we hung up the phone, I texted my best friend, 'Jeff just called! OMG he totally still loves me!' The second 'sending ...' appeared on my phone, I realized that I had sent that ridiculously cocky text to Jeff and not to my BFF. Lord help me."
—Our very own Debra Goldstein

The Mis-Text

A mis-text is every texter's worst nightmare! Sending juicy information to the one person whose eyes it wasn't meant for spells T-R-O-U-B-L-E. Before you go nuts and throw your cell out the window (like Deb wanted to after her monumental mis-text), take a deep breath, and know that even though this may seem like the most embarrassing thing ever, damage control is possible and just a text away.

In Debra's situation, she quickly bounced back and had no choice but to acknowledge her mis-text in the best way she knew how. Since both she and her ex-BF are movie buffs, she quickly retaliated with: "Uh, that was a movie quote!?" When he wrote back, "Passion of the Christ?" Deb knew she was back in safe territory. This fire was contained; however, she learned a tough lesson. At times when we're overcome with excitement, it's more likely that we can become careless with our texts. As caught up in the moment as you may be, it's always smart to double-check your text before sending.

Our grade school teachers said it best: "Remember to always double check your work before handing it in." It meant nothing to us then, but everything to us now. It seems like all technology these days gives you the ability to double-check your work before turning

texting tip

A Simple Solution to Avoid Mis-Texting

Send the really special BPTs to yourself first, ensuring they read correctly. Then copy and paste the text to the lucky lad and rest assured he got the message right.

it in. Voicemail lets you listen to the message you left, with the option of erasing it and starting over. Digital cameras allow you to look at photos immediately and decide if you want to re-shoot. Text messaging only sends messages when you are ready to send. You hold the power of pressing send. So make it your responsibility to double check your text, ensuring that all systems are go. Damage control is okay but prevention is best. Here are some proactive tips to avoid mis-texts:

Tips to Avoid Mis-Texting

- Proofread all VIP texts that would be considered risky if they fell into the wrong hands. ALWAYS check the name of the person who the message is going to before pressing send. It takes two seconds and can save much humiliation.
- Draft your important messages in another mailbox first. If you are worried about what to write and need to draft your text a few times before sending (which is totally normal), do so in a different mailbox. Disaster strikes if you accidentally press send and you send the draft message, "wanna go to the *fart* party?" when you meant to say, "wanna go the *frat* party?"
- Cell phones have spell check capabilities. Use this option when sending important texts. It's a small thing that can make a huge difference.

With cell phones getting smaller and technology more instantaneous, mis-texting has become all too common. Being aware of the possible mis-texting situations will help you become proactive and avoid social suicide. The last person you want to brag to about the details of your date last night is your date. Yikes.

Here are some mis-text examples plus damage control texts. Our best advice to you when a mis-text occurs is to own up to it quickly, find the humor in what happened, and pray for forgiveness.

Examples of Mis-Texts & Damage Control

Mis-text 1:

Text meant for your mom: (following first date with new guy) "Best date ever! Chris is a keeper. Get started on wedding invites!"

Sent to: Chris

This is the most common kind of mis-text. It happens because sometimes our fingers and brain cross messages. Therefore even though you meant to text your mom, you texted Chris, because clearly he was on your mind.

Damage control:

"Sorry meant for my mom. Who you will be meeting at our wedding. Next week work?" or

"Oops! Did you know that 1 in 7 texts you send are mis-texts? Looks like I got 6 more till my next:) P.S. I had a great time last night."

Mis-text 2:

Text meant for your BFF: "Guess what?! I went home with Dan last night! Call you later with the deets."

Sent to: Your boss, with the same name as your best friend.

Damage control:

"Scratch that! How embarrassing, totally meant for someone else. Hope this doesn't show up on my performance review!"or

"Oops, mistext! Well at least you know how my morning's going ;) See you at work!"

What Do You Do When You're on the Receiving End of a Mis-Text?

Mis-text 1:

Current guy you're dating texts: "You looked hot last night."

Sent to: You. Which is odd since you DIDN'T see him last night!!

Red flag! If your PBF texts you "You looked hot last night" and you spent last night at your parents' house, then *ding ding ding*, we have a problem. Go ahead and entertain the elaborate story he's sure to make up about how the second part of his text got cut off, which was ". . . in my dream. In my dream you looked hot last night." Unlikely. Trust your gut on this one. Looks like you just caught him red handed.

Damage control:

"I think you meant to send this to your other girlfriend" *or* "Funny, I don't recall seeing you last night. But yes I did look hot."

Try to remain calm, cool, and collected. Always come out with your head high in situations like this. He should be calling you right away to resolve his detrimental mis-text.

Mis-text 2:

Current guy you're dating texts: "I took Molly home and hooked up with her last night."

Sent to: You. Molly.

Damage control:

"She must have been wasted." *or* "Wow you're one lucky fella."

Even though you may be upset, find the humor in it since he's bragging. He obviously thinks you are a catch. Yes it's somewhat gossipy that he is texting his friend about your make-out sesh, but it's also a little flattering, no? Remember when John Travolta and Olivia Newton John's characters in *Grease* had way different reactions to their "Summer Lovin'"? She wailed about "staying out till 10 o'clock" while he made quips to his guys about "making out under the dock." Two very different sides of the story. Guys are cuddly and romantic with you and mean it, but need to show off in a macho way to their friends. Best to teasingly call him out on it and then let it go.

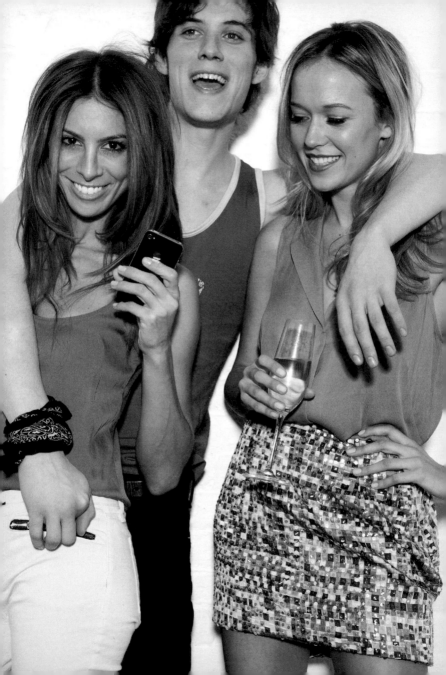

beyond
the basics

"I love flirtexting on BBM because it's very simple to use the 'end chat' feature and erase any trace of shadiness ever occurring from anyone else you may be dating." —Chris

WHEN FLIRTEXTING
IS CHEATING

Whether you're in an exclusive relationship or casually dating someone, you must be aware that flirtexting with other guys can create trouble in paradise. If you're in a committed relationship, any sort of playful text exchanges with guys other than your boyfriend are grounds for infidelity and will be held against you in the court of break-up. Even if you were only kidding around, flirtexting others while in a relationship can be hurtful, especially if exposed.

If you are single and flirtexting with many suitors there are guidelines to be followed if you're in the presence of other PBFs. There's truth to every text. Here you will find the guidelines for what constitutes texting as cheating according to your dating status.

If you're single and dating . . .

You're a flirt who loves having adoration coming from several directions, especially when it's in the presence of one guy without the other knowing. It's a contradicting feeling. It feels so right yet seems so wrong. After receiving Justin's text you instantly get a cocky little grin on your face that puts this air of confidence around you, which you wear quite well the rest of the night. Something about being with one guy while texting another gives you a small rush that you love. Being that you're not tied down in a relationship, you're pretty much a free agent who can trade up at any time. You've got a few fellas vying for your attention and you're running with it. And may we say, go you.

The private and instant nature that texting allows makes it so easy to flirt with tons of guys at the same time, it's a crime not to. As serial flirts, admittedly this is one of the features we like most about flirtexting. It's an easy way to keep dibs on all your PBFs within a finger's distance. However, let us be quick to remind you, it's also very possible that any of these guys you're flirtexting could be flirtexting other girls as well. Enjoy it and take it for what it's worth: harmless fun that creates a little excitement.

Guys deep down know that single girls have several guys they're talking to at once (because they do the same with several girls). They may know it, but they certainly don't want to hear it or actually see it. So be mindful of a few flirtextiquette rules if the occasion occurs while on a date:

Rules of the Two-Time Text
While Out on a Date

Don't leave your phone in plain view while on a date. Even though you're on a date with Jon but expecting a text from Jake, ensure your phone is placed in your bag and not on the table in plain view. Blinking red lights, vibrating sounds, and seeing messages pop up is distracting and will signal to your date that you've got better things to do than be there with him. Also, if you're not expecting a text from anyone, Murphy's Law will ensure when you're out on a date that other guy you like will finally text you. **Guys have a sixth sense and when you're out with someone else, they somehow feel the urge to contact you that very moment.** It happens all too often. Play it cool and stow the cell.

Don't check your phone in front of your date more than once. Unless you're ready to explain why you need to check your phone, don't do it, or be prepared to be called out on it. If you don't want to be confronted, check your phone when he's not around. It is understood you're going to check your phone once during the date. Checking your phone incessantly displays disinterest. If you're really into a guy you'll refrain from checking your phone until after the date.

Don't text in plain sight and assume he doesn't know who you're texting. If he sees you texting he will assume you're texting another guy. It's just how his mind works. But then again, we would probably guess the same if roles were reversed. It's hurtful and can be uncomfortable. In general, if you're going to flirtext others while around your date please be sure to do so discreetly. While he's away in the restroom or grabbing your coat, these are open invitations to text on the sly.

If you're having a sleepover, ensure your phone is turned off. If a guy is sleeping over and in the middle of the night your phone buzzes repeatedly with texts, expect uneasiness from your spooner. No one wants to hear your phone buzzing at 2 a.m. He knows it's not your mom. Checking your phone at night signals you're not interested, so check it in the morning. Most likely you'll both be doing the same thing.

If you're in a committed relationship …

Flirtexting other guys while you're in a committed relationship is not a light matter. Be it with an old boyfriend or someone new, flirty banter over text is not cool. Text is the written word. If anything, it is more real than if you say it to their face because it's traceable and able to be forwarded!

If your current beau finds out you've been flirtexting with another guy, more than just his feelings are going to get hurt. Use your best judgment and think through the consequences when responding to these texts. If you don't feel comfortable with your BF reading them, then you shouldn't be texting in the first place. Better to be safe than sorry.

The following are the guys who probably still text you even though you are in a relationship and tips on how to handle it:

Flirtexting an Old Boyfriend

Look, we know that you once had feelings for your old BF, and it feels good when he texts you out of the blue. However, getting in touch every once in a while is very different than text messaging every other day. Even if these flirtexts are platonic, it will still be very hurtful if your current boyfriend finds out. Using the silent treatment in this situation is universally known as a way to get out of verbally stating the obvious: that you're "with someone." He should take the hint and stop texting you. If he doesn't, then text him: "gonna have to call it quits with the flirtexting for now. The new guy might get jealous. I'll alert the press if things should change."

Flirtexting with Guy Friends with Whom You May Have Hooked Up With

These are the guys that fill up your little black book and who you probably flirtexted with before you were in a committed relationship. They come in and out of your life and check in every now and then. They could be aware that you have a boyfriend but that doesn't stop them from going after some attention from you via text. If they know you have a boyfriend and are still pursuing you, their attempts should be shot down. If they don't realize the degree of how "off-limits" you really are, make it clear and text: "Sorry, bud. You're a few months too late. I'm a taken girl now."

Flirtexting with a Guy Best Friend

This is tricky territory, as he is considered one of your friends, right? Boyfriends in general don't feel comfortable having you be so chummy and flirty with another straight guy. Even the most secure guy will still be on edge if this is the case. They know how their own minds work and assume this guy friend has more than "friends" on his mind. They may not be completely off. They may tell you they are cool with your friendship, but they still look at him as a potential threat to your relationship. We advise you take your boyfriend's feelings into consideration when sending flirtexts to your guy best friend. Even though he is your "friend" and sending suggestive flirtatious texts to one another is what you've always done, it's still grounds for jealousy and accusations of cheating. It's best to keep your responses as non-flirty as possible to avoid any problems. To set the record straight, try texting: "You know I love you but we've got to take a time-out with these flirtexts. I'm not in the market for a jealous boyfriend." Your best friend should understand because he wants what's best for you and therefore will respect your relationship. And, your boyfriend will continue to keep his mouth shut about your close relationship with another guy.

Recap!

That was a lot of information. To make sure you got it all, here's a quick recap of what NOT to do when flirtexting.

How to Lose a Guy in 10 Texts:

1. Over text
2. Use lots of symbols and smiley faces
3. Send heavy, emotional texts
4. Mistext
5. Respond back right away
6. Drunk text/ LNBT
7. Misspell everything
8. Send unoriginal, generic texts
9. Wait too long before responding
10. Text in front of your date

"My flirtexting has dramatically decreased since getting engaged. My flirtexts now consist of messages like, 'Babe, do you want me to pick up a chicken for dinner?' Although I'm fairly certain that turns her on." —Scott

HOW TO SPICE UP A RELATIONSHIP THROUGH TEXT

If you are reading this chapter it means that you have successfully passed through the early stages of flirtexting and into a fabulous committed relationship. Congratulations are in order! Just because you have entered into the land of "we" does not mean that you can call up your cell phone provider and cancel your unlimited texting plan. Flirtexting is still fantastically important in an existing relationship—now you're able to take it one step further.

In a relationship, the fact that you both care deeply about each other is out in the open and felt equally by both parties. This commitment allows you the luxury to relax a bit more when sending texts. You don't have to spend as much time on your BPTs and you can go ahead and throw texting timelines out the window! Whew. Flirtexting in a relationship opens the door for you to explore the other, shall we say, more *risqué* things you can do with text. With that, feel free to text things that only prove how into him you are by *going beyond the flirtext.*

Sexting

"I love flirtexting because I can
pretend my junk is 3 inches longer
than it is. The girl won't find out
the truth until it's too late." —Ross

When you've been with the same person for a while, what better way to spice up your relationship than with a fiery flirtext? One that will arouse more than just his senses (wink wink). Yes, that's right. We're talking about sexting, and it's a long-term dating DO.

Sexting: Descriptive sexual conversations through text with the intention of arousing the person on the receiving end.

When the mood strikes, you can reveal fantasies and sexy thoughts to him while he is out of town, at work, or even across the dinner table. There's always time for a fantasy text!

Sexting Examples

- While the two of you are at dinner with friends, text him that if he casually uses the word "wet," or any funny/sexual word, in conversation at least six times before dessert comes, then you'll do that thing he loves later.
- When you're at dinner and he gets up to use the restroom, text him "did I mention I'm not wearing any underwear?" (even if you are). He'll be asking for the check before you order your main course.

- If he's on a business trip and you miss him, text "I'm all alone in this big bed of mine. What should I do?" Believe us, he'll gladly take it from there!

- If your man plays sports and you are at his game, text "Score now and I'll let you score with me later ;)" or "Win or lose, you're scoring with me tonight ;)." If he checks his phone during halftime, watch as he runs faster, hits harder, and throws further during the second half. If he doesn't get the message until after, he'll still appreciate the flattering gesture, win or lose.

- If he asks you, "Want to go to a baseball game?" respond with, "Sure, but only if we can go to third base ;)" OR if he says, "Basketball game tonight?" you say, "Are you insinuating foul play? Love to."

Tips on Sexting the Right Way

- To avoid your friends or co-workers seeing sexy texts or photos, delete them immediately from your phone after sending.

- If someone asks you to send a sext and you're uncomfortable doing it but still want to please them, try the funny approach and take a picture of your elbow and send it with a text reading "Guess what body part this is from?" OR, grab a Victoria Secret catalog and snap a pic of one of the girls and say "Here you go."

- With sexting, the motto is "less is more." If you reveal everything in a text message, then what does he have to look forward to?

Long-Distance Relationships

Sexting is especially beneficial in long-distance relationships. The need for sexting heightens when you're not around one another. It's an excellent way to remain close, especially if there's a time difference. If you are getting ready for bed on the East Coast and he is finishing up a meeting on the West Coast, he is still able to connect with you in your time of need. Sure, it's not the real deal, but hey, it beats nothing at all! (Um, did we mention this is a great form of safe sex?) Texting helps make long distance more bearable by having the ability to be in constant contact.

Virgin to sexting? Not to worry. It doesn't hurt. Talk about that thing he did to you last night that you loved or what you want to do to him when you see him next. Talk about how your salad came with a really big cucumber and you thought of him. Be bold, be blunt, and be bad. Be a little selfish when you dirty text and say things that will turn you on in the meantime. Chances are if it turns you on, it'll turn him on twice over.

Shy by nature? This is a great way for those of you on the shyer side to let your man know what you like sexually. If you are too embarrassed to tell him in person, use text and the casual, safe environment that it provides to tell him your fantasies. You'll be surprised how much you will benefit from being open about your likes and dislikes through sexting.

Not into sexting? Flirtexting with your man doesn't always have to be dirty. Texts like suggesting pizza and football for a Monday night date or randomly sending "I love you" go a long way, too. Long-term relationships can get mundane. You've constantly got to be doing little things to keep the sparks alive. Sending a random, thoughtful flirtext is a great way to show him how much you care.

- Randomly text, "I love you" or, "I'm crazy about you." It's simple, it's quick, and it will make him smile.
- Send a recent sports fact about his favorite player like, "Linsanity is on tonight!"
- If he's having a rough day at the office, suggest a date night including his favorite things and tell him about it to get him through to the five o' clock whistle. "Agenda for the evening: cooking your favorite dish and watching the Knicks game. See you at 6."

With technology these days, the sexting possibilities are endless. Imagine what you can do if your cell phone had a camera on it. Oh, but wait … it does.

Photo Text

Ah, the infamous photo text. Now that most cell phones have cameras in them, sexting has risen to a whole new level. All those scandalous things you're texting your man can now include illustrations and pictures.

Men are visual creatures. They'd much rather see what you are wearing than for you to tell them. Therefore, we understand the enthusiasm that guys are overcome with when it comes to the camera phone.

> *Guys can lose their heads, and their phones sometimes, and we don't want to see your boobs on the internet.*

Whenever you are taking a racy photo text of yourself, proceed with caution. Never include your face in the photo. Even though you are in love now, what happens if something goes terribly wrong and you have a nasty break-up later? You guessed it! Hello, Facebook photo tagged of you and your large breasts! May we remind you that you're also "friends" with your boss?

Here are a few classy ways of using the photo text to spice up an existing relationship:

- Never include your face in a naked photo text. This protects you from embarrassment if the photo falls into the wrong hands.
- Take a picture of you sticking your head out of the shower, showing some sexy shoulder or your smooth leg, and write, "can you get me a towel?" or "bath time would be soo much more fun with you...."
- Take a picture of your bed—or better yet, you in it—and write "room for two," or, "Can you meet me here later?"
- If you bought some new lingerie and are planning on wearing it that night, take a picture of the lingerie still in the bag and text "I bought you a present ... if you're a good boy, I'll give it to you later." He'll be so excited he'll be on his best behavior.

- Send a snapshot of your lips, with a message that reads "they miss you."
- If he's begging for you to take a sexy picture of yourself to send him, take a picture of your friends cleavage or a girl's in a magazine and write, "Not mine, but I'm still thinking of you;)"
- If you're on a beach and missing your man, snap a pic of you in your hot bikini and write, "wish you were here" in the sand.

A Warning About the Photo Text

If you are NOT in a serious relationship with a guy and you text him dirty photos of yourself, he will forward them to his friends. We can't stress enough how you must proceed with caution when sending racy photos of yourself. Be smart, ladies, and trust us on this one. Guys can be pigs sometimes. The last thing they

The most important thing to remember when using text to spice up an existing relationship is to do a little bit of everything. Send him dirty ones when you're feeling a little feisty, fun and playful texts when you're thinking about him throughout the day, and intimate flirtexts when you miss him. The key is to mix all these different kinds of spices together. This will keep him on his toes and wanting you more and more with every flirtext sent.

texting tip

are thinking about when they receive a hot photo of a *new* girl they are dating are her feelings. We've seen too many of our girlfriends get hurt because they sent nude pictures of themselves to guys they were "just dating" to find out they've become the screensaver on his friends' phones. This is why we only advocate sending these kinds of texts when you are in a committed relationship. Otherwise, expect what you send to him to be forwarded to his entire soccer team.

Pre-Packaged Texts

Since we know you're busy, on-the-go women, we took the liberty of listing some BPTs to guys' most common flirtexts. Like us, they are mood dependent. The content of our text will depend on many things: the time he sent it, how sincere it was, and whether or not we're having a good hair day.

These pre-approved and ready–to–use flirtexts are sure to get the response you want and then some. By the way, feel free to take all the credit for them. It's what best friends are for.

Added bonus: We asked all of our hot guy friends to tell us what they *really* mean when they text these things. Their candid and truthful answers are written verbatim, under "what it means."

1. His text: "Hi"—and nothing else.

What it means: He's basically saying, "I'm here, don't forget about me..."

If you're feeling	Respond like this
Flirty	"Hey handsome"
Sassy	"Try again" (Calling him out on his lame attempt).
LOL	"Who is this? Uncle Leo?"(Classic *Seinfeld* quote. Guys love *Seinfeld*).
Straight to the Point	"Hey u what's happening?"
Jane	"Heyyyy"(A pointless response to his pointless text . . . and mind your y's).

2. His text: "What are you up to tonight?"

What it means: He's beating around the bush and wants to ask you out. He's hoping you are free and will wait to see what you're doing before asking.

If you're feeling	Respond like this
Flirty	"Not sure. What'd you have in mind Mr. Party Planner?" (Ball's back in his court … where it should be!)
Sassy	"Ridiculously busy. Need to update my Facebook profile. You?"
LOL	"I don't know. Was thinking about going to Home Depot. Buy some wallpaper, some flooring. Then maybe Bed, Bath, & Beyond. U?" (Never hurts to quote *Old School*)
Straight to the Point	"You tell me." (He's blushing)
Jane	"No plans" (Social suicide, ladies!! Always have plans even if you are sitting at home watching Lifetime with zit cream on. He doesn't know that!)

3. When you want to see him that night and he's not flir-texting!

What it means: He's either really busy or not that into you. (Fingers crossed for really busy.) Don't fret, he could be having a moment of insecurity/loneliness/vulnerability and will text you in the near future. However, this isn't always the case. You should begin to explore other options.

If you're feeling	Respond like this
Flirty	"I know a really cute [insert your hair color here] who will be at _____tonight. U should stop by and check her out."
Sassy	"[Insert your plans here] tonight. Get involved."
LOL	"People I want to see tonight, for 400 please. Answer: Who is [insert full name of recipient]?"
Straight to the Point	"Plans tonight? Buy you a milkshake?" (What guy in his ice cream-loving mind would turn this down!?)
Jane	"Hey!! What are you doing later?" (Lame. Too generic. Boring. Need we say more?)

4. *When you've been texting back and forth all day and suddenly he stops texting, leaving you hanging … Text one of these to get a quick response.*

What it means: See Scenario 3.

If you're feeling	Respond like this
Flirty	"I'm not sure I like your attitude."
Sassy	"Plans tonight? Buy you a milkshake?" (What guy in his ice cream-loving mind would turn this down!?)
LOL	"Are we playing the quiet game? Because if we are, you're really good at it!"
Straight to the Point	Re-send your last text and act like your phone is messed up.
Jane	"Are you ignoring me?" (Again, a case of social suicide.)

5. *When he name drops and instantly turns you off.*
   His text: "Hey going to [insert latest hotspot] tonight.
   [Insert name of C-list celeb] is going to be there.
   You should come."

What it means: HE'S A TOOL. He thinks you're a cool chick and feels the need to impress you in order to compensate for his low self-esteem. Or, he thinks you are superficial and can pick off the low-hanging fruit with some materialistic bait.

If you're feeling	Respond like this
Flirty	"Wow I didn't realize who I was dealing with ... you're kind of a big deal huh?"
Sassy	"Who's that?" (This will put him in his place.)
LOL	"Hang on I think you dropped something. Oh never mind, it was just those names."
Straight to the Point	IGNORE his lame attempt to woo you through who he knows. Hopefully he'll get the hint when you don't respond and try a second attempt, with a lot more class.
Jane	"I'd love to meet _____ sometime. I'm such a huge fan!"

6. His text: "Are you still mad at me?""

What it means: He f'd up and knows you are pissed off. Either you are ignoring him or he is afraid that if he calls, you will blow up again. He's texting to test the waters first. Depending on your response, he'll know how much he can get away with in the future.

If you're feeling	Respond like this
Flirty	"Depends. How are your groveling skills?" (Say this when you're no longer mad, but just want to give him a hard time.)
Sassy	"Who is this? Lose my number." (Obviously you're still mad.)
LOL	"Ask me again in 5 minutes." (Keep doing this until he gets annoyed and calls. Something he should have done in the first place.)
Straight to the Point	Don't respond. He will get the hint.
Jane	"No. I could never stay mad at you! <3" (If you say this, he'll do whatever he did to piss you off again. Guaranteed.) *or* "Yeah im mad. It was really disrespectful and I cant believe u would do that to me." (Don't have "feelings" talks over text.)

7. *His text:* When he's been flirtexting you off the chain and you want him to call.

What it means: This may be a problem. Or, he may think you prefer to communicate non-verbally. Drop a hint that you are not one of those girls and see if he responds in kind.

If you're feeling	Respond like this
Flirty	"This is crazy. Here's my number. Call me, maybe?" (Thanks Carly Rae Jepsen for supplying us with flirtexting fodder!)
Sassy	"FYI—Unlike Verizon, I don't offer unlimited texting plans. Feel free to call anytime to discuss updating your service. We have a special going on now."
LOL	"Just heard the craziest thing. Did you know these texting devices also place phone calls? We should really be more adventurous with our phones."
Straight to the Point	"I'm running to the gym [or out to dinner]. Call me later." (Being the first one to end the conversation is the best way to leave him wanting more. If he likes you, he'll follow up on that call later.)

| Jane | "I really wish you would call me instead of texting." (Don't put him on the spot. This sounds needy and eager. Both turnoffs.) |

8. His text: "When do I get to see you again?"

What it means: He wants to see you.

If you're feeling	Respond like this
Flirty	"I don't know. You tell me."
Sassy	"Depends. Were you thinking coral diving in Malaysia or more along the lines of dinner and a movie?"
LOL	"When Ashton Kutcher goes to space. Oh … shit. I'll be ready at 8." (Any improbable pop culture related news feed will work here.)
Straight to the Point	"When you make reservations."
Jane	"How's tonight?"

9. You invite him to hang. His text: "Maybe I'll meet up later."

What it means: It's noncommittal.

If you're feeling	Respond like this
Flirty	"Hope so."
Sassy	"Sounds promising."
LOL	"Maybe I'll already be in a relationship by the time you get here."
Straight to the Point	"Cool, would love to see you."
Jane	"I feel like you don't want to see me." (Seriously, Jane. Work with us girl.)

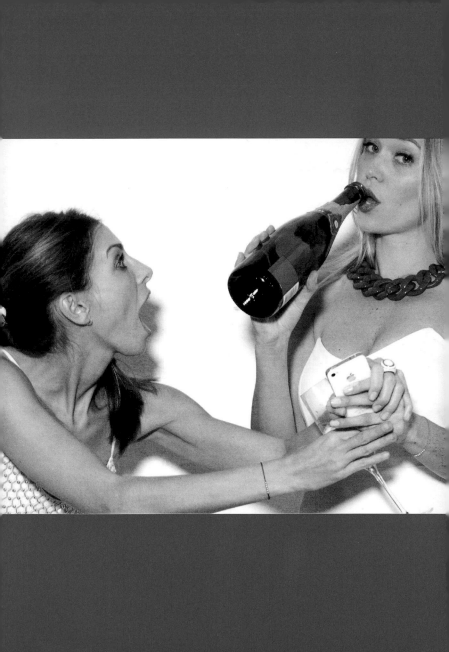

digital dating

"Guys totally stalk girls' Facebook pages. I obviously don't, but I've seen my friends do it."

—Alex, Facebook Stalker

FINDING LOVE ON FACEBOOK

Facebook is awesome. It's a social tool that allows us to casually connect and innocently "stalk" our family, friends and acquaintances. It informs us when our camp friends get engaged, which of our high school friends have babies, and when our sorority sister goes on *The Bachelor*. No need to attend awkward reunions just for that information, simply log-on to your news feed and you'll be all caught up. In today's dating world, Facebook has made things "complicated." Never before have singles been able to so easily reconnect with their past, strengthen a connection with someone they just met, or reach out to a stranger with common interests.

For the single girl, Facebook is essential. It's chock full of valuable information about potential suitors, current lovers, and ex-boyfriends. The same girl who "googled" her date five years ago, now does her due diligence on Facebook. Google is great, but most likely it won't tell you that your crush is a great snowboarder (hot) or what

texting tell-all

Deb's Facebook Love Story

Have you ever had a guy send you a friend request that you think looks familiar, but you just can't remember why, or if you've even met? You "accept," because he's friends with a few of your friends, but then don't hear from him until maybe a year later when he sends a private message asking you out. Well, that guy turned out to be my last boyfriend. So you might want to think twice before hitting "not now," you never know where love may find you.

his ex-girlfriend looks like. All vital and valuable information a girl should know. So if you're single and have Internet access, then jumping on the Facebook bandwagon is simply one request you cannot "Ignore."

10 Things You Need to Know About Facebook & Dating

1. If a guy leaves without asking for your number, rest assured if he liked what he saw, you'll receive a Facebook friend request from him in the near future.

2. Searching through your friends' photo albums for hot guys is an efficient way to look for love.

3. Finding out if your crush is attending that party Friday night is easy with event RSVPs.

4. Blind dates . . . what are those? Thanks to Facebook, blind dates no longer exist.

5. Profile pictures are a saving grace when you met someone at night and want to know what they look like during the day.

6. Facebook makes rejecting people easy. A simple click on the phrase "not now" does the dirty work for you.

7. Getting the scoop on a new crush from your mutual friends is a must before agreeing to a date.

8. Facebook is the best way to reunite with an old high school flame.

9. Facebook kindly alerts you when your crush goes from "In-a-Relationship" to "Single."

10 . Thanks to Facebook reminders, you'll never forget his birthday again.

Facebook has revolutionized the way we connect and date today. It has opened the door to a world where we no longer have to go to the same school, be in the same bar, or even live in the same state to start a relationship. Who would have guessed a dorky kid from Harvard would be the one to make online dating cool? Liv, that's who. She knew all along . . .

texting tell-all

I was attending Boston University in 2004, around the same time Mark Zuckerberg started Facebook at Harvard. I signed up just when it became available to the Boston schools. All my friends looked at me like I was nuts not to be on MySpace instead, but I knew this was better. I even sent Mark a friend request in hopes of connecting with the inventor. Needless to say, I'm still patiently waiting for him to accept. It's the least he can do for an early adapter.

—Olivia, Facebook member #911,013

Facebook Profiles 101

> "When I get a friend request from a girl,
> I look at her pictures first, and only accept
> her if she's hot." —Luke

Today, not only do we judge a crush by his flirtext, but we judge him by his Facebook profile too. How many times have you been excited about a guy you just met, or someone your friends wanted to set you up with, just to be let down when you saw his Facebook page and were turned off by his profile? News flash ladies, judging someone by their Facebook profile is a two-way street. Therefore, knowing what to include and what to exclude from your page is crucial if you want to come across looking like the perfect catch.

Creating the Perfect
Facebook Profile

1. Always use a photo showing a clear view of your face with good lighting—no back of the head shots, pictures of you wearing sunglasses, or images of you from far away. Save the artistic shots for your albums.

2. Make sure your profile picture is of you solo. Pictures with friends are sweet, but you run the risk of him mistaking you for your BFF who your arm is around.

3. Don't include photos where you're dancing on tables, holding a shot glass, or doing anything questionable that mom, your boss, or your potential husband might be turned off by. While you may think your party pictures make you look "cool" and "social," others may peg you as a "party girl" and "immature." Instead, include pictures that tell a well-rounded story. Pictures of you at a sporting event, on vacation, or spending time with friends and family, show that you're a well rounded woman with lots of interests and good values.

4. Don't overdo the "about yourself" section. We've said it once and we'll say it again, less is more ladies! Remember this when you're listing your top 20 favorite movies and TV shows. *Our rule-of-thumb is to include no more than three options for each category on your profile.* Anything beyond that divulges too much information, and could open his eyes to unnecessary deal breakers before you even get a chance to meet.

A Tip for Posting a Successful Profile Picture

Having a profile picture that you clearly took of yourself in a bikini with puckered lips, believe it or not can be detrimental to your social life. If you think that photo will attract the type of men who want to take you home to meet mom, think again.

The key to having an alluring profile is to tell a story through pictures and interests that speaks honestly about who you are, and doesn't reveal everything upfront, so you keep some mystery intact.

5. Make sure your relationship status is set to no status until you're married. We can't stress this enough. Telling the world you're in a relationship now might seem like a good idea, but changing it three times a year makes you look non-committal.

Facebook Dos and Don'ts to Live By

Dos

1. *Do* set the "sharing" feature on your other social applications to private. If you have applications like Twitter, Spotify, Pinterest or Foursquare linked to your Facebook account, make sure you turn "off"

the share feature, so your friends aren't alerted every time you listen to "Someone Like You" by Adele, pin something onto your wedding board, or check-in to "Wax Everything."

2. *Do* limit yourself to one hour a day on Facebook (this includes your Facebook cell phone app). Digging on Facebook for an extended period of time can lead to the FOMOs (fear of missing out) and feelings of envy.

3. *Do* change your profile picture once every six months to a year, so people know your account is active.

4. *Do* respect status updates and limit posting to no more than 3 to 5 times a week. We don't care if you just ran into Lady Gaga at the grocery store, if you already hit your limit this week, call your friends to tell them.

5. *Do* be truthful in your profile. If you say you like skateboarding and run marathons, make sure you can back that up

6. *Do* use appropriate language. No one wants to date a girl with the mouth of a truck-driver, no matter how hot she is.

7. *Do* keep photos of yourself to a minimum. No one wants to see 100 photos of you solo and only two of your friends and family. It makes you look self-absorbed.

8. *Do* be wary of the Fan pages you join. Even if joining "Ingrown Toenails" is a joke, no one else knows that. (Yes, this group really exists.)

Don'ts

1. ***Don't*** change your Facebook profile picture every week. Doing so makes you look vain.

2. ***Don't*** friend your ex-boyfriend just to spy on him. It will become addicting and drive you crazy.

3. ***Don't*** overpost on your crush's wall—doing so puts you at high risk of pissing him and lots of other girls off.

4. ***Don't*** be that girl who "likes" every photo two seconds after it gets posted. It makes you look like you have too much time on your hands.

5. ***Don't*** post status updates for the sake of posting. Your 1,300 friends don't care that you changed your nail color to "Braziliant."

6. ***Don't*** poke people. It was annoying in Kindergarten and it is still annoying now.

7. ***Don't*** come on too strong by sending unsolicited sexy photos of yourself.

8. ***Don't*** post status updates about a guy you are dating or used to date. Whether it's a nice or snarky comment, it only speaks ill of your character.

The Rules for Single Girls & Facebook

"When a girl private messages me, she wants to hook up. End of story." —Peter

I'm single. What are the rules for "friending" mutual guy friends I think are cute?

Friending mutual guy friends is OK in moderation. Some guys like it, some think it's aggressive, but the overall consensus is that they find it flattering and know exactly what you're doing. Don't go

> *If you're single and friending guys you've never met (even if they are mutual friends), they are going to assume you think they're cute and want to date.*

overboard and start friending every guy that pops up in your "people you may know" feed, but sending a friend request to a hottie here and there is completely fine.

What are the rules for sending the guy I just friended a private message?

This move is a bit more aggressive than just sending a friend request. If you "friend" a guy and he thinks you're cute, chances are he'll end up messaging you first, which is just what you wanted! But when you "friend" him and private message him first, he might be a little turned off by how forward you are. This doesn't mean he won't entertain the idea of dating you, just be careful what you say in your message. We suggest opening with something like, "I think we met once at (name of random party). You were that guy who (insert funny memory here)."

According to our friend Jason, "When a girl private messages me, it doesn't matter what she says, it means she wants to hook up. 'I love the pictures from your trip I want to hear all about it . . . *over dinner before we have sex.*' See what I mean?

How should I set my privacy settings if I'm open to meeting someone on Facebook?

> "Don't have a profile that's set to private. Facebook is for stalking." —Tom

Facebook allows you to choose how viewable you want certain albums or photos to be. We highly suggest setting your privacy so that most all of your information and photos are available to "friends" only, but if you're single and open to meeting someone on Facebook, then we recommend leaving one album viewable to "friends of friends." Make sure the photos in this album are edited for the eye of a potential suitor, so they'll be enticed to friend you and see more!

Digital Break-Ups

> "It's pretty obvious when a girl just broke up with someone because her Facebook page becomes much more active. It's a good way to let me know she's single and ready to mingle . . . with me I hope." —Chase

Chances are, after a break-up, stalking your ex's Facebook page will pretty much become your M.O. for the next couple of months. You'll assume every woman he befriends is his new girlfriend, cry when pictures of him are posted with girls in his vicinity, and follow his trail of comments to see if it leads to clues revealing that he cheated on you. Now we know this is just *Jane* coming out in our time of despair, which is why it's important to understand all of these things will only prolong the healing process.

Facebook is a double-edged sword. It's great for finding love, but not so fun when that love fizzles out, and we find ourselves having to breakup twice: once in real life and once digitally (detag!). Knowing the appropriate amount of time to wait before changing your relationship status, the rules are for deleting your ex's friends on Facebook, and if it's okay to detag yourself

Stop, *Block* & Roll

We've all either thought about it or gone through with blocking an ex-boyfriend, current crush, or in some cases, current boyfriend from Facebook. This happens when the weak, insecure girl in all of us (say hello, Jane), takes over and persuades us do things we normally would never do.

Here are some of the reasons you probably blocked or dropped him from FB:

1. He did something really annoying that pissed you off
2. He didn't pay you enough attention
3. A combination of 1 and 2
4. You became obsessed with looking at his page and the only way to stop was to block him
5. You're being shady and don't want him to see the pictures of your new boyfriend on your page

from photos of you and your ex, are all things we must consider when going our separate ways. We now have to cut our ex's out of our digital worlds as well as our real ones. But how do we do that?

Tips for Digital Break-Ups

Is it rude to delete my ex from Facebook?

If you can't stop looking at your ex's profile page and spend the better part of your day analyzing all the new activity on it, then yes, delete him immediately. But the best thing to do is to emit self-restraint. We know, easier said than done! If that's impossible, then the next best thing is to be honest. Tell him you're going through a hard time with the break-up and are deleting him from all forms of social media for the time being. Then, take a deep breath, swallow your pride, and defriend. Telling him you're doing this looks a lot better than deleting him out of spite. This will save you hours of agonizing over new girls he friends in the future.

When is it okay to change my status back to single?

Whether you were the dumper or the dumpee, don't change your relationship status or detag photos before you've even finished having the breakup conversation. It's insensitive, immature, and shows you're hurting. Take the high road and follows these rules for when it's appropriate to de-couple yourself on Facebook.

If You Dated:
- 3 months, you can change your status the next day, post breakup
- Less than a year, wait about 3–5 days post breakup

- 1–2 years, wait about a week
- Over 2 years, wait about 1–2 weeks

What are the rules for deleting his friends?

If you had a bad break-up and want him effaced from your life completely, then delete all mutual friends and don't look back. If your break-up was amicable and you like his friends (especially that one you met at his soccer game), then keep them for the time being. No need to shun a PBF down the road just because your current one happens to be on the outs!

> "When my friend's girlfriend broke up with him, he emailed all his friends asking us to defriend her. We all thought that was super lame. We're adults, and we are not doing that." —David

Managing the Status Quo

Remember the time when your friends found out you were dating someone naturally, instead of through a status update sent to a bazillion of your friends? Well that's still the way we like to roll, which is why we strongly recommend having **no relationship status** on Facebook until you're married. This will deflect any unnecessary drama down the road. If it's too late and you've already changed your status to "In-a-relationship," the appropriate time to change it will depend on how long you date, and how amicable the break-up is.

Is it okay to untag yourself from photos with your ex?

Yes, just do so subtly. Don't feel the need to delete all images of the two of you in one fell swoop. Doing so can make you look bitter. However, if you're at the point where you're starting to date other people, then make sure photos of your ex are removed. Otherwise it will look like you're still holding on to your ex.

If You're in a Relationship…

If you're in a relationship and a guy private messages you to ask you out, what's the proper thing to do?

If a mutual friend sends you a complimentary messages and asks you out, feel free to thank him for the offer, and quickly let him know you're in a relationship. Seeing that you have friends in common, it's best not to burn any bridges. Otherwise, ignore any cheesy, unsolicited pickups from strangers. Keep in mind, you always run the chance of your boyfriend using your computer to log onto his Facebook account and accidentally signing automatically onto yours. Don't put it past him to peek, as we are sure you would too.

If you're in a relationship, should you de-friend your ex's? Also, is it OK to keep communicating with them via private message?

You do not need to de-friend your ex just because you found a new boyfriend. However, it's best to cut off any casual chit-chat with your ex via text, email and Facebook. Unless you have something specific you need to discuss with them, avoid the whole "whats up" conversations, just to be safe.

Turn-Ons, Turn-Offs, & Dirty Little Secrets

Facebook Turn Offs:

- "I hate when a girl over posts on my page. It's like she's peeing on me to mark her territory. It's super annoying." —Sebastian
- "Bad profile pictures or lack of pictures. Girls love pictures. Pretty girls love pictures even more. If you don't have a lot of pictures and you're a girl, you're hiding something." —James
- "When girls post about how amazing the weather is where they are. I get it. Weather sucks in New York." —Rich
- "When a girl doesn't accept my friend request and instead relegates me to 'Awaiting Approval' purgatory forever. Ew. Bitch." —Seth
- "Girls who over post on my wall—that gets annoying." —Evan
- "It's super unattractive when girls post pictures of themselves out five nights a week at different clubs. I don't want to date someone who goes out every night. Get a day job." —Zac

- "Posting photos of yourself in a bikini on a private jet or yacht that belongs to middle-aged men you're "friends with." —Jon
- "Making kissy faces and posing with your hand on your hip because you think it makes you look slimmer." —Max

Facebook Turn Ons:

- "When a girl talks shit about football every Sunday and knows what she's talking about." —Luke
- "A profile that at the very least attempts to create the image of a wholesome, attractive, charming, classy, ambitious, and educated young woman." —Jake
- "A great profile picture." —Andrew
- "A great Spotify playlist that introduces me to cool, new bands." —Keith
- "Photos of skinny girls chowing down on a burger are hot." —Justin
- "Those black and white photo booth shots make girls look hot." —Jon

What's your go-to Facebook move that works every time?

- "Do we know each other?" —Dan

Facebook secrets, facts, truths, confessions girls should know:

- "Sex is the only thing that the website is good for. If I were married, I'd definitely delete my account." —Seth
- "When girls post tons of pictures of themselves

all done up hanging over other guys after a break-up, I think it's completely transparent and the most ridiculous thing ever. You're obviously going out of your way to make me jealous and it makes you look stupid. Guys will sit there and laugh at it. It's almost like 'I win.'" —Ric

- "The first thing I do when I add a new girl to Facebook is look for albums titled Vegas, Hamptons, or Miami. You know you're going to see girls in slutty outfits or bikinis in these pictures, and if there's an album titled "Halloween," you know you're getting a combo of both." —Justin

- "I used to have a FB app that actually tracked who visited your profile, how often, etc. That was actually incredible. Only a handful of people knew it existed. So no one was prepared for it. The results, however, were surprising. It was never who I would've expected to FB stalk me. It would always be the kind of quiet, yet cute (and possibly sexy) girl who gave me the cold shoulder in real life. She would be the one visiting my page 6–10 times a day. Anyways, it gave a lot of extra ammunition for when I would run into those girls and they'd act like they weren't interested." —Jack

"In online dating having the freedom to choose who you really want to date doesn't guarantee a successful match, but at least you've got nobody to blame but yourself." —Greg

TOO GOOD FOR
ONLINE DATING?
THINK AGAIN

et's face it. While getting a date has never been your
problem (hair flip), you recently noticed a decline in
your current dating pool, as friends have started pair-
ing up and settling down. While the thought of online
dating has definitely crossed your mind—after all, it
worked for your entire book club—you still have your
doubts. You thought online dating was for people who
had trouble getting a date, and would rather stay in and
watch Ryan Gosling movies than post a public dating
profile for the whole world to see.

If it was up to us, Prince Charming would have landed
on our doorstep at the ripe age of five. If we could only
look into the future and know that before we're eighty
we'll be happily married, we'd be able to enjoy the
dating process so much more. Unfortunately psychics
are unreliable and we're stuck combing our friend's
Facebook pages for eligible bachelors to friend. But

what happens when you've tapped out all of those resources? Online dating, that's what, and lucky for us, it's no longer a last resort!

According to a recent study, there are over 40 million Americans using online dating. (That's a lot of PBF's looking for love online!) Between Facebook, Twitter, Pinterest, Spotify and Instagram, we spend so much of our social life online already, it's no surprise the web has become a popular place for singles to meet. If you're into meeting guys at bars, at dinner with friends, or at the gym, then online dating is really no different. More Americans have opened themselves up to online dating and it's about time you do too.

With the increase of cool new dating websites today, online dating has attracted a fresh pool of normal, successful, viable dating options for the modern woman. Your idea that dating websites are a place for creepy predators with mustaches to stalk their prey or where the beautifully challenged go to date, is outdated and quite frankly not true. From musicians to doctors to ivy-league educated bankers, online dating is the new hotspot and getting in is easy.

Not only is online dating a great option for people who work really late and often don't have time to make it to every dinner or party to which they're invited to, going online gives you a much broader range of eligible guys to choose from. You know that every guy on there is single and looking to meet someone; you never have to worry about talking to a guy who is already in a relationship or not ready to be in one. Not to mention you're given access to various social circles you may never have encountered previously.

Before you start your online dating adventure, check out our tips and advice gathered from our personal experience and knowledge of online dating, as well as the experience of our friends who have all jumped on the online dating bandwagon. In this chapter, you'll learn how to set up a compelling profile, how to read between the lines of his private message, which dating site is right for you, and much more.

The Dos and Don'ts
of Online Dating

"I have no trouble meeting new guys or getting a date, but I still use online dating as a way to meet even more guys and go on even more dates. What can I say, I'm a friendly girl." —Debra

Dos

1. *Do recognize your profile picture is the #1 most important thing.* Make sure your profile picture actually looks like you. Posting a professional headshot where the angle makes you resemble a Kardashian sister will just lead to disappointment.

2. *Do use online dating for target practice.* Think of online dating as a sport—use it to sharpen your dating skills and to find out what you're looking for in a long-term partner.

3. ***Do read into profile names.*** Names like Namasteguy, HangTenBen, LakrSfan and Soxnundies, can help you determine someone's interests quickly, ex: these guys are into yoga, surfing, the Lakers, and well . . . you get the idea.

4. ***Do be original and thoughtful with your email greeting.*** Avoid sending universal messages like, "Hey how are you?" and "What's up." Instead, say something that will strike conversation right away like, "Where were you in your profile picture?"

5. ***Do be wary of recycled pick-up lines.*** "You're the first girl I've reached out to on this site, so don't let me down!" and "I enjoyed reading your profile. We have a lot in common . . ." are all recycled lines.

6. ***Do some fact-finding before meeting up.*** Before you agree to go out with a guy, get his email address so you can look him up on Facebook. If you have any friends in common, interrogate them and get the scoop.

dating tip

You can usually tell right away which guys are serious about online dating and which are just looking for a good time. If his first email to you includes his number, an invitation to meet up, or a list of your sexy body parts, you've got a player on your hands. Proceed with caution.

7. ***Do play it safe.*** If you do agree to a date, tell your friend where you're going and when you'll be back. That way if he kidnaps you, she'll know who did it: CraZy4U911.

8. ***Do choose one well-tailored date per week.*** By focusing on one date per week, you avoid getting restless man syndrome, where you're never satisfied with your dates because you're always curious who's right around the corner.

9. ***Do send private messages at acceptable times of the day.*** The best time to send or respond to a private message is during the weekday or around dinner time, or on Sunday afternoons. Avoid messaging late-night on weekends as guys look at time stamps and will think you're sitting at home, alone on a Saturday night.

And Some Don'ts

1. ***Don't spend more than 20 minutes a day searching for love online.*** With so many eligible guys online, be careful not to sabotage your actual social life by staying home on your computer instead of going out with friends.

2. ***Don't mobile date solo.*** If you're using a GPS dating app like MeetMoi, Skout or Speeddate, make sure you have a friend or two in tow. These apps allow you to see who's in your neighborhood to make meetups spontaneous. But it can also potentially be dangerous, so use it wisely.

3. ***Don't join a dating website and expect the hotties to flood your inbox.*** The reality is that every guy who messages you may not be the prince you're looking for. Be ready to pull your sleeves up do some digging of your own to find the guy that suit your taste and lifestyle the best.

What Guys Mean When They Say...

He says . . .	Translation
He describes himself as a "snuggler."	Get ready to be read poems and be doted on, he's sensitive.
"I've been told I'm very handsome."	Probably by his mother. He will spend more time getting ready than you.
He's an "Entrepreneur/ Actor."	He's "self-employed" and most likely lives with his parents.
He says he "loves to laugh."	He's funny and you better be too.
He doesn't fill out his height.	He's under 5'5".
He says he "loves long walks on the beach."	His dates lack imagination so be prepared for cheesy champagne and strawberry-filled nights.

He says . . .	Translation
"Football is my passion."	He'll live on the couch on Sundays.
"Once upon a time, I went through an intense bodybuilding phase, but now I hit the gym as more of a social activity to connect with friends."	He's chubby.
He mentions his "mom" at least once in his profile.	You'll always be #2.
His list of favorite movies includes all of Will Farrell's greatest hits.	He's hasn't picked up a book in a while.
He uses emoticons and drops LOLs a lot.	He's trying to compensate for his lack of the funny genes.
"Looking for a girl who is fun with no drama."	He's got some awesome ex-gf stories.

Twitter, Words with Friends, & Other Tech-Savvy Ways to Meet

"Last summer this cute guy asked me out, but I was dating someone else at the time. A year later when I got my iPhone, I sent a request to my friend (with the same name) to play a game of "Words with Friends" via my iPhone app. For the first three days, I didn't realize I was actually playing an intense game with the guy who asked me out! He started IM'ing me to catch up through WWF's IM, and eventually asked me out via WWF messenger. We're now dating and I always tell him it was his impressive vocab skills that really did it for me."

—Melissa

"I met Seth briefly at a tech event and decided to start following his interesting thoughts on twitter, along with a dozen other colleagues I met that day. I noticed right away how drawn I was to Seth's tweets, whether they were about a band we both liked or a current event upon which he had an opinion. One might say I was "sweet on his tweets." One day, I replied to one of his tweets. This initiated a twitter chat, which led to text messaging, which led to a date, which most recently led to a proposal!"

—Nicole

Which Dating Website Is Right for You?

With over 1,500 online dating websites today, the big question is—which site is right for you? This section breaks down some of today's most popular dating websites to help you decide where your Mr. Right is waiting.

Match.com

The Men: Smart, fun, cool, and normal. Think football playing prom king or those really hot guys in beer commercials with a little bit of scruff wearing a plaid shirt.

Tip: When in doubt try Match.com first.

Profile: Generic questionnaire, not too intimidating, about 40 minutes to set up.

Cost: Fee to join/pay to engage/$17 per month for a six month membership.

Celebrity Most Likely to Be a Member: Ryan Gosling

EHarmony.com

The Men: Straight-laced, marriage-minded, on the fast track to getting engaged.

Tip: Older demographic, average dater being 35+.

Profile: Extensive questionnaire, expect to spend 2 to 3 hours on it.

Cost: Pay to join/$30 per month for a six month membership.

Celebrity Most Likely to Be a Member: John Krasinski

HowAboutWe.com

The Men: Young, hip, new to online dating.

Tip: Try their mobile app. It's easy and fun to use.

Profile: Low-maintenance where you suggest date ideas as a way to meet people.

Cost: Free to join/pay to engage/$15 per month for six months.
Celebrity Most Likely to Be a Member: Bruno Mars

JDate.com
The Men: Funny and normal. Lots of lawyers, doctors, and grad students.
Tip: You don't have to be Jewish to be on this website.
Profile: Generic questionnaire, 30 minutes to an hour to set up.
Cost: Free to join/pay to engage/$25 per month for a six month membership.
Celebrity Most Likely to Be a Member: Shia Labeouf

OKCupid.com
The Men: Casual, cool and creative.
Tip: Great blog with infographics showing clever and hilarious insights based on user interactions.
Profile: Low maintenance.
Cost: Free.
Celebrity Most Likely to Be a Member: James Franco

PlentyOfFish.com
The Men: Diverse and eager to date/hook up. Not so much marriage material.
Tip: Has a MeetMe feature that allows you to view locals.
Profile: Low maintenance.
Cost: Free.
Celebrity Most Likely to Be a Member: Vinny from *Jersey Shore*

The Best Way to Online Date

If you're one of those girls who signed up for online dating with a fake name and profile picture just to see what it's like, you're not alone. Lots of girls do that to test the water (guilty!), which is why we created DatingShotgun. com as a way to help girls dip their toes into online dating before taking the plunge.

> **DatingShotgun.com** **A free, weekly email featuring a curated selection of the top eligible bachelors in your area, who are currently online dating. No public profiles, no fees, just a great way to see who is on which site before deciding where to commit.**

"The best profiles tell a story, like when a girl writes, 'All you need to know about me you can learn from what I did last weekend . . .' and she proceeds to write about her adventures in dog walking and her run-in with extremely spicy tuna."
—Anonymous hot online dating guy

How to Create an Attention-Grabbing Profile

The process of creating a superb online dating profile requires a bit of self-promotion which is awkward. Think about it. If your friend introduced you to her single boss, and the first thing he said was, "Hi! I'm an attractive, successful, witty guy who loves working out and traveling," you'd run the other way! Growing up, we were taught bragging about ourselves is an unattractive trait, so why then is it okay for us to do it in our online dating profiles? The answer is, it's not.

Your dating profile is your first impression in online dating. This is why it's important your profile reflects who you are in a way that will attract the right men and ward off the wrong ones. This, my friends, is easier said than done.

Here's what your average, 5'5, good-looking girl's dating profile says: "I'm an outgoing, driven, successful, genuine, young woman with an open mind and a big heart. I'm equally comfortable dressing up in a cocktail dress or relaxing in a t-shirt and jeans. On the weekends I love going to Pilates, hanging with friends and family, or watching football (Go Patriots!). I'm looking to meet a wonderful man, who makes me laugh, shares my same interests, and is not afraid to fall in love."

She seems sweet. Problem is there are thousands (if not millions) of dating profiles with some version of this same exact paragraph. The guys we interviewed who online date all said the girls they message are ones with interesting and captivating profiles. That's why your profile needs to be awesome and stick out. Here's what you need to do.

Top 5 Tips for Creating a Captivating Dating Profile

1. **Write in lists.** He's skimming hundreds of profiles so by listing your traits, likes and dislikes, you have a better chance of him actually reading what you wrote.

dating tell-all

"My online dating profile says I like guys who can quote movies for days. Now I have an inbox full of guys trying to woo me with their best movie line! As it turns out, seeing what they quote actually says a lot about them. One really cute guy said he loves quoting Woody Allen and French films. I knew right away that was never going to work." —Deb

2. *Give guys an easy opening to strike up a conversation.* For instance, if you say "I'm really into learning how to surfing," expect the sexy surfer to message you offering private lessons.

3. *Opt for interesting facts describing who you are rather than generic adjectives.* This informative and fun list should imply you're easy-going, genuine, sarcastic, and open-minded without blatantly saying it.

4. *When in doubt, leave it out.* Reveal just enough information to pique his interest so he inquires about more. If you go overboard with your likes and dislikes, you run the risk of turning him off before he actually gets to know you.

5. *Be honest.* It's a waste of time and money if your profile is fiction. Trust that if you've done a good job of describing who you are and what you're looking for, the right guy will take notice.

An example of a great online dating profile and why it works:

- I love productive Saturdays and sleeping in on Sundays. *(Shows you're motivated when you need to be but you also know how to relax.)*
- I'm a Yankees fan with a vast knowledge of useless baseball trivia. *(Great opening for sports lovers to send messages with lots of trivia questions.)*
- I have a soft spot for Salmon Sashimi w/ spicy mayo. *(Invites to his favorite sushi spot to follow.)*
- I'm really good at Words with Friends and play more often than I should. *(Shows you're smart and tech savvy. Open invite for guys to test your vocab skills by challenging you to a game.)*
- A few of my fav's: Pulp Fiction, It's Always Sunny in Philadelphia, Jay-Z, Jon Stewart, Dan Brown, red wine, Barcelona, yoga. *(Shows you're well*

The Good, the Bad, & the Lame

The good thing about online dating is you're able to tell who the jerks are right away. Since online dating is a platform for self-indulgence, guys who only care about status, money and looks will tell you so in their "About Me" section. Example: "What can I say, I'm the real deal. I'm attractive, intelligent, successful, witty, well-traveled, I have a great job and I'm fun to hang out with."
—Modest212, online dater

rounded with lots of interests. Chances are he's into one of these as well, offering the perfect opening to share his favorite Dan Brown book or Spanish wine recommendation.)

- I'm looking for a guy who laughs at all my jokes and isn't afraid to wear pink. *(Shows you have a good sense of humor, are sarcastic, and like a guy with confidence.)*

The Male Perspective on Dating Profile Pics

- Photos are most important. You have to be able to see their face. No pictures of you wearing sunglasses or from far away, and you have to include a full body shot or the guy will think you're hiding something. Guys need to know what they're getting themselves into.
- Photos of girls with other guys or when girls post lots of pictures of themselves in exotic locations are lame. It's too obvious they want me to know they're well traveled.
- Include at least one photo of you dressed up. It doesn't have to be at a wedding, but a photo of you at a formal event shows that you clean up nicely.
- There's nothing wrong with a tasteful beach shot, but make sure you're on a beach! If you're in your apartment wearing a bikini, then that's kind of desperate.
- Guys don't like photos of girls being super goofy. Meaning no pictures of you at a deli trying to eat

a giant salami hanging from the ceiling. That's not funny or attractive.

- Be selective of photos of you with children. If it's a picture of you at a kid's birthday party with lots of other kids around, then I'll assume it's a niece or nephew. But if it's a picture of you holding a three-year-old toddler in your lap, I'll wonder if you're a single mom.
- Certain things freak me out a little, like when a girl has a photo that is too sexy, where she's lying on her bed with a 'come hither' look.

Q & A With A Hot, Male, Online Dater

What's your biggest online dating turnoff?

Unoriginality. Can't stand when a girl says, "I'm kind, caring, and just love to laugh and love a guy who likes to laugh at himself." Ugh, shoot me.

What are your biggest online dating turn-ons?

Being real, great photos, creativity and humor. I love when a girl writes anything original, even if it's off the wall and if I don't quite get it. It still tells me something about her and shows her personality. For example: "I'm addicted to eating Bibimbap at this little Korean restaurant in the East Village near my house. It's ridiculously spicy and I have to drink a slushy afterwards, but it's totally worth it!"

The first connection I made on Match was with a woman I dated for six months. Her headline said she was the queen of sarcasm and the rest of her profile was refreshingly honest. I liked that a lot.

What's a tip for girls when creating profiles?
I like it when girls quote movies.

What are your thoughts when a girl reaches out to you first, instead of you reaching out to her?
I don't mind when girls reach out to me. It's happened a few times and I've had good dates. It depends on what they write. If they go overboard and send me a really long message then it makes me wonder. One girl wrote, "I saw your photos and I thought you were gorgeous." That's weird. If a girl says something in the middle, that shows she looked at my profile and then calls me out on something funny, then that's cool.

Do you care what time a girl sends you a message?
Girls should be mindful when they send private messages. I always look at the timestamp and if it was sent at 2am I think it's weird. If it was sent on a Friday or Saturday night, then I picture her sitting home, alone, watching Love Actually. Not a good look.

What's an online dating secret?
I've got two approaches that work well, but surprisingly one works better than the other. The first is the natural approach—I'm funny, mention something in her profile I can relate to, and at times say something random, just to add in a filter to see how she responds. That works a lot of the time, but sometimes girls think it's strange. The second approach is to keep it brief and not reveal too much in your message. For instance, "Hey there, I really enjoyed reading your profile. I saw that you've been to India. I went once and found it really interesting. Write back if you're interested and let's grab a drink sometime." Ironically this works a lot of the time.

....

He Sparked My *Pinterest*

There's something to be said for photo-sharing apps, like Instagram and Pinterest, and the dating world. Recently I was looking at who my followers were on Pinterest, and I noticed this guy who I'm distant friends with, not only followed my boards, but he "liked" and repinned some of my pins. As nerdy as this may sound, in the digital world when someone "repins" your pin, it's flattering. Even if it didn't originally come from you. It's like a digital compliment, if you will.

This made me curious about my distant friend, and I wondered if we had more in common than I had originally thought. So, I lollygagged over to his Pinterest page and what I found was essentially a snapshot of this life in the form of a photo journal. By looking at his boards, I was able to learn about his taste in *architecture and interior design* (good to know in case we ever move in together), what his *inspirations* are (my man's got to have goals), where he wants to *travel* (also good to know incase he surprises me with a trip for our anniversary), and what his taste in *fashion* is like (note: if he has too many pins in this board perhaps he's not the man for you, or any other girl). I was pleasantly surprised at the amount I learned from looking at his boards, and felt like he was definitely a person I'd like to get to know more.

What happened next, you ask? I went back to my list of followers to see if any other cute, single guys were following me, and checked out their boards. Then, I went back to his boards and repined a picture he posted that I liked. Hopefully he'll reciprocate with an invitation to join him at the five star resort in Croatia I posted on my travel board. Fingers crossed.

If you're in a relationship, use Pinterest to give (or get) hints to your significant other about what you want for your birthday! Guys usually need a bit of help in this department. If you really want to make it easy for him, create a board that's called, "My Birthday Wish List" and I'm pretty sure he'll take the hint!   —Deb

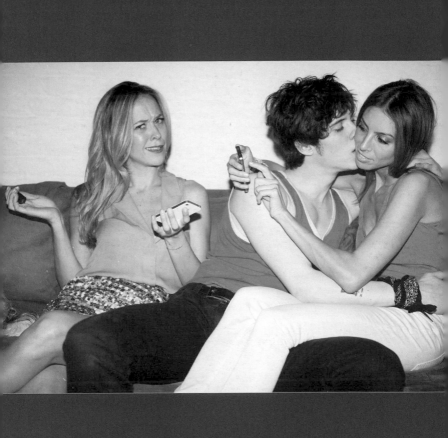

bonus features

"If you want a response, comedy is always a good bet." —Nat

MOVIE QUOTES

Crush: Party at Matt's house tonight. You in?
You: No. I've got my little sister's dance recital to go to.
Crush: Lame.
You: You better lock it up!
Crush: No, you lock it up!

We're not sure why, but guys love to quote. A movie, TV show, comedian, you name it. If someone else said it, they'll quote it. At times, we've even seen guys speak to one another solely in quotes, a phenomenon that can be rather annoying. But for some reason they seem to think it's hilarious. To be honest, we think it's pretty funny, too. There's nothing sexier than a guy with a great sense of humor, and if he's quoting funny movies, we betcha he falls under that category.

Guys like movie quotes and find nothing hotter than to receive one via text from a girl they are crushing. When used properly, movie quotes are a fantastic way to respond to his flirtext. Text messaging with boys is all about the *zingers*. Movie quotes combine the power of wit and useless knowledge and are sure to spark tons of intrigue from the lucky lad on the receiving end. Be it an old school movie or today's blockbuster hit, catchy, clever movie quotes all quickly assimilate into an average boy's daily banter. So when you fire back with a line from his favorite movie, watch as your dating stock rises.

Oh, and did we mention it's a surefire way to grab his attention, especially if he's been MIA recently? Boys have told us that when a girl nails a movie quote, it's super impressive and piques their interest even more. They get as much of a reaction, if not more, than that hook-line-sinker-fish move they go crazy for on the dance floor.

The appeal of movie quotes is exponential. Now, let us teach you a few tips on how to use them over text. Follow these rules and use some of our examples below and he'll be uttering "Here's looking at you, kid" in no time.

dating tip

Best Case Senario

You quote without using quotation marks, he gets it, and quotes back from that same movie. If you want to keep going with it and need more lines from that movie, just go online. IMDB.com has tons of quotes from every movie ever made. You can keep this dialogue going for hours of useless fun.

1. *Follow our adage: When in doubt, quote.* If he's not texting/calling you and you are thinking about him but have nothing of substance to say, instead of just writing "Hi," write a movie quote. What's more appealing to a man than a snappy one-liner taken out of his favorite blockbuster? Not much besides the fact it's coming from you, missy!

2. *Ensure the timing of a movie quote makes sense and is therefore aligned with your deliverance.* Be sure that your timing is appropriate for sending the quote. If used in the wrong context, he might not get it and your attempt could backfire. Which means, "Houston, we've got a problem." Best time to flirtext a quote is when you recently saw the movie together or were recently discussing a movie you both like. Same goes for TV shows that are both your favorites and a new episode just aired.

3. *A word to the wise: be tactful with your quotes.* Just because boys love them that doesn't mean you should be throwing them around left and right. *Don't* overdo the quoting because it'll lead him to say "Hasta la vista, baby" and then we'll be saying, "Welcome to Dumpville ... population, you." Catch our drift?

4. *When in doubt, use quotation marks.* We recommend texting your quote without using quotation marks around it. It's funnier that way. But if you think he might not get it, then go ahead and throw those suckers around your quote.

Here are some guy-friendly quotes that are pretty safe to use no matter what the circumstance. Take note that you don't have to use the whole quote every time. Just pull from it what you need that makes the most sense in that situation.

Great Movie & TV Quote Texts

Argument

Use these when you are arguing with him and need some fighting words:

- "Erroneous! Erroneous on both counts!"
  —Wedding Crashers

- "Let me tell you a little story about a man named 'Shhh'."
  —Austin Powers

- "This is one doodle that can't be undid, homeskillet."
  —Juno

- "I'm not your buddy, friend."
  —South Park

- "Agree to disagree. When in Rome."
  —Anchorman

- "Hi, I'm Earth. Have we met?"
  —Tommy Boy

- "Put a cork in it, Zane."
  —Zoolander

- "Break yo'self fool."
  —Superbad

Attention Grabbers

Use when you want to say hello, but don't want to just write "hi":

- **Your text:** "It smells like updog in here."
  Him: "What's up dog?"
  You: "Oh, nothing much, what's up with you?"

  —The Office

- "Bueller? Bueller? Bueller?"

  —Ferris Bueller's Day Off

- "I don't know how to put this but I'm kind of a big deal."

  —Anchorman

- "Hey Peter. What's happening?"

  —Office Space

- "I've been performing feats of strength all morning."

  —Seinfeld (Frank Costanza)

Great Random Quotes

Use when you need a great response back to his random text:

- "That's what she said."

  —The Office

- "I got to get outta here, pronto. I got a stage five clinger. Stage five, virgin, clinger."

  —Wedding Crashers

- *"Mortal Kombat* for the Sega Genesis is the best game ever."

  —Billy Madison

- "First rule of Fight Club: You do not talk about Fight Club."

  —Fight Club

- "The greatest trick the devil ever pulled was convincing the world he didn't exist."

  —The Usual Suspects

- "Do you ever get down on your knees and thank God you know me and have access to my dementia?"

  —Seinfeld (George Costanza)

- "Don't forget to bring a towel."

  —South Park

- "Looking at cleavage is like looking at the sun. You don't stare at it, you get a sense of it and then you look away."

  —Seinfeld (Jerry)

- "Funny, she doesn't look Druish."

  —Spaceballs

- "I've negotiated my butt off, Giorgio."

  —Zoolander

- "Who is this? Uncle Leo?"

  —Seinfeld

- "Night is a very dark time for me."

  —Blades of Glory

Words of Encouragement

Use when he needs a little pick-me-up:

- "You're on the rebound. You're like an injured young fawn who's been nursed back to health and is finally going to be released back into the wilderness."

  —Old School

- "What are you going to do for an encore? Walk on water?"

  —Wedding Crashers

- "I'm sick of following my dreams. I'm just gonna ask where they are going, and hook up with them later."

  —Mitch Hedberg (a super funny comedian)

- "My advice to you … is to start drinking heavily."

  Animal House

- "We got no food, no jobs, and our pets' heads are falling off!"

  —Dumb and Dumber

- "You stay classy, San Diego."

  —Anchorman

- Elaine: "Ugh I hate people." Jerry: "Yeah they're the worst."

  —Seinfeld

Weather Reference

Use when he asks you how the weather is:

- "It's so damn hot. Milk was a bad choice."

    —Anchorman

- "I'm sweatin' like a Tijuana whore!"

    —The Break-Up

- "It's too damn hot for a penguin just to be walking around!"

    —Billy Madison

Feeling Sick

Use when he asks how you are feeling:

- "I've got a fever and the only prescription is more cowbell."

    —SNL

- "I think I've got a case of the black lung, pop."

    —Zoolander

Travel/Airport

Use when one of you is traveling:

- "Why you going to the airport? Flying somewhere?"

    —Dumb and Dumber

- "I'll be back before you can say blueberry pie."

    —Pulp Fiction

- "May the Schwartz be with you."

    —Spaceballs

- "Are we there yet are we there yet are we there yet"

    —The Simpsons

- "There's no reason to become alarmed, and we hope you'll enjoy the rest of your flight. By the way, is there anyone on board who knows how to fly a plane?"

—Airplane

Calling Him Out

Use when he is getting on your nerves and you want to give him a hard time:

- "I'd like to be cowboys from Arizona or pimps from Oakland but it's not Halloween. Grow up Peter Pan, Count Chocula."

—Wedding Crashers

- "It's such a shame. You're so money and you don't even know it."

—Swingers

- "Just when I thought you couldn't get any dumber, you go and do something like this and totally redeem yourself!"

—Dumb and Dumber

- "You think that you are too cool for school, but I have a newsflash for you, Walter Cronkite... you aren't."

—Zoolander

- "Fat drunk and stupid is no way to go through life, son."

—Animal House

Admitting Fault

Use when you messed up and want to acknowledge it:

- "I'm sorry I called you a hillbilly. I don't even know what that means."

  —Wedding Crashers

- "SAMSONITE! I was way off. "

  —Dumb and Dumber

- "Damnit Derek, I'm a coal miner, not a professional film or television actor."

  —Zoolander

Asking Him Out

Use when you want to see him and want him to know it:

- "Tower, this is Ghost Rider requesting a flyby."

  —Top Gun

- "I'll be in the neighborhood later on, and I was wondering if maybe you wanted to get some frozen yogurt, or perhaps a whole meal of food, if that would be agreeable."

  —Old School

"Because in a digital age,
you should be able to get
your digital groove on." —Keith

TEXT LINGO

Remember when "TGIF" was the only acronym you knew? Good times. Today, it's nothing out of the ordinary to shorten our words in order to save time and much needed space. Our busy lives have affected our language as well as the way we communicate. Proper English has transformed itself into abbreviations, acronyms, and slang. Through texting, we've officially created an unofficial new lingo.

The language of text consists of short, abbreviated letters and numbers, combined with complete words. Text messaging allows for only 160 characters per text message. Since this is a limited amount of space to work with, wireless users created a language to accommodate text messages. Below is a glossary for common texting lingo as well as some hip new terms we use in our everyday lives. Feel free to spread the word....

P.S. Our list is limited because we do not recommend going crazy with the abbreviations. Boys get turned off if girls use too many of them in a flirtext. But we urge you to adapt these and text away with your best girl friends. They are meant to be fun supplements to your texting conversations, not to be taken seriously. Just avoid looking like you spend too much time with your ten-year-old sister is all we're saying.

P.P.S. We wanted to note that a texting abbreviation longer than five characters long is not an abbreviation—it's just ridiculous. No one understands what you are talking about, and you run the risk of looking foolish. Don't do it. Below we've listed a few of these ridiculous abbreviations that prove our point:

AWGTHTGTTA: Are we going to have to go through this again?

ROTFLOLAPIMP: Rolling on the floor laughing out loud and peeing in my pants

MTFBWU: May the force be with you

Flirtexting Glossary

<3 Love or heart

Besos Means "kisses" in Spanish. An alternative to "xoxo" when signing off.

BF Boyfriend or current crush

BFF Best friend forever

BFFAE Best friend forever and ever

BPT (Best Possible Text) A formula created by sending just the right text, at just the right moment, to get you exactly what you want. These are the type of flirtexts you should always be sending to your PBF.

ciao Can be a greeting or sign-off; means both hello and goodbye in Italian.

Cheers A British signoff.

Dreamy The new "cool."

Epic Something that's a huge deal or great.

F2F Face to face

FBF Favorite boyfriend. This is the boyfriend that you liked the most, maybe even loved. We don't just throw this phrase around. There can only be one of these.

French Smooch, kiss, anything involving a little harmless tongue action.

G1 Good one!

G2G or **GTG** Got to go

GF Girlfriend

Goss Gossip

KMA Kiss my ass

LNBT Late Night Booty Text; a flirtext sent anytime past 10 PM asking you what you're doing. These are purely sexual.

LOML Love of my life

Lylas Love ya like a sister

Mental Better than amazing. Example: "Um, did u see my new Louboutin's ? They're mental!!"

NBD No big deal!

Neat The word we use when we're bored with what you're telling us. Example: Boy: "I make over 500K a year and drive a Mercedes and have a house in Miami … " You: "Neat." (You may or may not want to also roll your eyes here.)

PBF Potential boyfriend

PIBE Play it by ear.

QT Quality time

SOL Shit out of luck

SOS The international distress signal meaning "Save our Ship." We use it to signify "Help me."

SS Social Suicide. Example: Mis-texting your current crush (instead of your BFF) that you think his brother is hotter than he is would be total SS!

TS Texting Sponsor

THX *or* **TY** Thank you

TMI Too much information

TTYL Talk to you later

TUI Texting Under the Influence

Vintage Referring to someone you consider way too old to date, or a reference to old news. Example: "Ryan is hot, he's just way too vintage for me."

Word Multiple meanings: for sure, I agree, absolutely. Example: Boy: "Meet me at my place at nine?" You: "Word"

WTD What's the deal?

WTF What the f*ck!

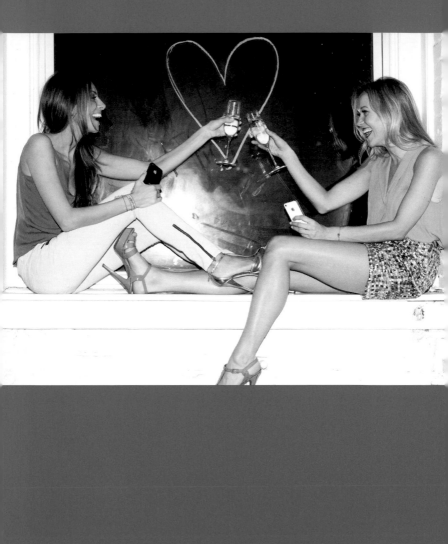

ACKNOWLEDGMENTS

We want to express our deepest gratitude and a very special thank you to Michael Goldstein (aka "Dad-ager") for your generous support, sound advice and for being so darn optimistic. Not only do we feel lucky and grateful to have you on our team, but you've helped us grow into savvy business women, and we thank you for that.

A loving thanks to Olivia's mom, Anna Kripp, for her love, immeasurable support and for always pointing out when an eyebrow needs tweezing. And to Liv's little brother, Peter Baniuszewicz. How lucky am I to have such a loving brother who still teases me? Love ya.

To Deb's mom, Fern Goldstein, for leading by example and being the kind of woman I hope to turn into one day. Your love, support and patience are immeasurable. And Deb's sister, Rebecca Shomair.

Thank you for your support, connections, and Friday night dinners. Love you.

To our legal super hero, Darrell Miller, whose extreme care and belief in us is one of the driving forces that keeps us going. We strive to make you proud. Thank you for always guiding and guarding our opportunities.

To the brilliant and talented E. Jean Carroll, we're so honored to have the woman whose words we live by open-up our book. If it weren't for your column in *ELLE*, we'd be thrice divorced by now.

A major shout-out to boyfriend/lawyer extraordinaire, Keith Pollock for his pointed advice and loyal support. Thank you for being so understanding when Olivia needs to join an online dating website or two for "research." Lots of love.

A special thanks to Sarah Dickman, the Nicholas Ellison Agency, and everyone at Skyhorse Publishing for believing in Flirtexting before it became the "cool" thing to do.

Thanks to our best friend Jason Levine. (Yesss.)

Big thank you to these fellas for no reason at all (wink, wink): Richard Jefferson, Scott Peiken, Josh Green, Nat McCormick, Eric Richman, Jake Avnet, Eric Larson, Josh Capilouto, John Del Cecato, Ross Cooper, Chris Candland, and Gene Kansas.

A huge thank you to Ryan Stratton, Chris Berkenkamp, Melissa Baer, Shawn Sachs, Nick Godfrey, Keith Esernio, Brooke German, and Marco Bollinger for donating your time, expertise, and services to us in exchange for flirtexts, dinners, and friendship. We really appreciate you guys, and all that jazz.

Thanks to our amazing and gorgeous girlfriends, for generously allowing us to poke around their love lives (knowing we might expose them in our book!), and for always standing by us: Nisha Bhagat, Jenna Caine, Courtney Parks, Hillary Tuck, Candice Taylor, Erica Winograd, Anna Klein, Renee Belluomini, Lauren Whritenour, and Janie Dim.

Thanks to our Nosara crew. Let's get loooose.

Notes